Paul Colver

P AUL C OLVER

The Aging Reversal Course

ISBN: 1439262128
ISBN-13: 9781439262122

contents

Preface

Aging Reversal Research

In our culture spry 90 year olds are often viewed as curious anomalies—even as freaks of nature—while in fact these vibrant people are normal in the truest sense of the word. True, they may have 'good genes' but their lives are invariably the result of a properly cared for physiology—something each of us can learn to do for ourselves. To see a delightfully fit, 88 year old go to youtube. http://www.youtube.com/watch?v=fY79KbCptTo

Even after substantial research in support of aging reversal most of the world is still bemoaning the misguided notion that at certain ages the body will deteriorate into a state of disrepair similar to that of everyone else in their age group. There is no lack of research to refute this misguided thinking: simply google 'aging reversal', or indeed, many individuals have regained lost vitality and youthfulness.

THE GOOD NEWS

The good news is that to return to youthfulness we only need to discover the balance our unique physiology requires and then learn how to create and maintain this balance. We can be spry and youthful at any age, and our body, being self interested, is highly motivated to help.

What is needed, and what *The Aging Reversal Course* provides, is an enjoyable, time-proven program for maintaining and, if necessary, re-introducing balance and subsequently vigor and zest into our physiology.

THE COURSE

The Aging Reversal Course is not about renunciation and struggle and suffering coupled with a diet of gruel and grey slop for breakfast, lunch and dinner. It is not about 'no pain, no gain'. On the contrary, the focus is on the enjoyment and the pleasure of living.

I hope the words 'enjoyment' and 'pleasure' jumped off the page at you. The proper understanding of being satisfied and sensuality is essential to aging reversal. As we will see pleasant, sensual living results in youthfulness; stressful misuse of the senses ages the body.

The course begins with sessions on effective breathing and hydration. Then suitable diet, weight management and exercise, as well as daily, seasonal and lifetime routines are established **based on individual requirements**. With an understanding of how to satisfy the body's needs in place the later sessions present physiology's most powerful means for reversing aging.

Have Fun

An individual may have good results working solo through *The Aging Reversal Course* but I recommend taking the course with a companion or with a group. Laughing along with others is fun and the group will provide added insight.

MY WISHES FOR THE READERS

My first wish is that you seize this chance to create the health you deserve. Once the zest and energy begin to flow you will want more of it. Enjoy!

Second, I hope you spread the good news. The understanding of human physiology presented in **The Aging Reversal Course** has the power to create change. Humankind is waking up! People are recognizing their uniqueness and taking responsibility and control of their well being. Please forward this good news to your friends.

KUDOS

My heartfelt thanks go out to the people who have supported me in writing this course: To my son Ben Colver for his insightful comments and work as a wordsmith; to my daughter Ellie Colver Metcalfe for her thought provoking questions, and encouragement.

Many thanks to the friends and readers too numerous to mention: Darlene Holt, Elizabeth Innes, Ray Harris, Anna Novikov, Garda Rowe, Janet Dalgetty, Everett Marwood, Elle Magne among them.

Thanks also to the editors, illustrators, and computer wizard Dianne Anstey, and all who helped with the huge challenge of getting the book into print.

Thanks also to photographer Yvonne Lein of Parksville, British Columbia.

My thanks also go out to the experts in the field of Ayurveda, other Eastern approaches to health, and the teachers of Indigenous Medicine. Making available their understanding of human physiology is indeed a great gift for the world family.

Introduction

THE BODY REBUILT

Our skin, liver, the eyes, nearly all of the body is constantly being rebuilt. Most of the body is less than 2 years in age; much of it less than 2 months old, and much of it—the stomach lining for example—is rebuilt daily. How and why do we age?

Ayurveda has some novel answers regarding aging and also some novel means to ameliorate and reverse it. Aging, in part, according to Ayurveda, is the result of the body's cells losing their 'memory' and forgetting how to rebuild themselves properly. *The Aging Reversal Course* reviews some of the reasons why cells lose this intelligence, but to be time effective the focus is on what is required in order to re-enliven the body's memory in order to rebuild itself accurately—that is to say, to recreate youthfulness.

Ayurveda

Cognized and written down thousands of years ago in what is today India, Ayurveda presents a unique understanding of the workings of human physiology, and as we will see, is much in sync with the recent findings of Quantum Physics. In brief, the main concepts of Ayurveda are that our body is equipped with built in intelligence. An intelligence that automatically directs the rebuilding of the body, and secondly intelligence that calls out for what is required in order to accomplish this prodigious task. This intelligence is not the mysterious stuff of the twilight zone but as we will experience beginning early in the first session, intelligence that may be readily accessed to create a more youthful physiology.

The Aging Reversal **Course** does not adhere to any particular 'school' of Ayurveda. Nor is it an amalgam of the various current thinking regarding Ayurveda; nor is it an attempt to present a comprehensive study of Ayurveda. As the title suggests the course is primarily concerned with aging reversal. While Ayurveda is considered as a tool to promote youthfulness, Tai Chi, concepts from Chinese Medicine and Indiginous Medical Practices are also considered. From study and life experience *The Aging Reversal* **Course** is based on **the author's current understanding of how individuals may satisfy, in a Life supporting manner, according to the intelligence found within their body, the requirements of their unique physiology.**

A RADICALLY DIFFERENT APPROACH TO LIFE

The Eastern approach to life is often inaccurately portrayed as one of renunciation and suffering. Monasticism, though touted by the monks who practice it as the best and only path, is not a life suited for the 'householder'. In his introduction to *The Yoga Sutras of Patanjali: A New Translation and Commentary,* the author concludes his thoughts regarding the folly of renunciation with the terse line: "… properly understood, (the eastern approach to life) is not a system of giving up life, it is a system of adding to life."

Supporting this view is Vasistha's instructions to Rama found in the great Vedic treatise _Vasistha's Yoga_. "To the ignorant, this body is the source of suffering; but to the enlightened man, this body is the source of infinite delight." **_Session 13: The Purpose of Sensuality_** makes clear that while unbridled sensuality is a waste of Life energy; proper use of sensuality is essential to better health and aging reversal.

EASTERN AND INDIGENOUS HEALING SYSTEMS BEGIN WITH AN ALTERNATE VIEW OF LIFE:

- Our body performs trillions of function per second in order for us to thrive. The body is our ally, not our enemy.
- Health care is not an arsenal of weaponry for combating the body but instead a storehouse of protocols for supporting the body in its incredible feats of healing.
- If the body loses the knowledge of how to rebuild itself there ways to 'recalibrate' the systems within us in order that proper rebuilding takes place.

These concepts are a welcome relief from the "No pain, no gain" delusion of a culture largely out of sync with reality.

SOMETHING FOR EVERYONE

What is it you seek? Breathing techniques for better oxygenation? Soft silky skin? Better assimilation of water and nutrients? Techniques to deal with cravings? Better endurance? Uber-fitness? Proper nutrition? Exercise that transports you effortlessly into the Zone? Weight management? Flexibility? Strength? An understanding of human physiology? A better understanding of your own unique physiology? **The Aging Reversal Course** has answers.

WHAT TO EXPECT

The early sessions of the course (regarding oxygenation, hydration, nutrition and proper digestion) are a preparation for the middle sessions which focus on peak performance and euphoria through Vedic Exercise.

Session 6: Understanding Physiology includes a questionnaire to assist in understanding your unique physiology. In the next sessions, diet, spice mixes for cooking, and daily routine are considered in relation to specific needs of individual body types.

The latter sessions present the importance of the Gap, Life, and Consciousness as seen in the light of the poetry of William Blake and the findings of Quantum Physics during the last decade of the 20th century.

- That we have sensuality is not an accident: but there is a need to understand how to best use and enjoy sensuality.
- That we can 'dip into silence' and experience great joy and bliss, is also not an accident. There is a need to understand why we are built as we are, and how to make the best use of these gifts.

Let's proceed to **Session 1** which deals with properly oxygenating the body and provides initial insight into the concept that the body has intelligence.

Session 1
Effective Breathing

Sailing, skiing, flying a kite: how wonderful to spend a day in fresh air, to return home purified, fresh and full of Life. Plenty of oxygen and the release of accumulated toxins are wonderful for our well being. Let's learn what information the body has for us regarding proper breathing.

BREATHING EXERCISE 1: DETERMINING PROPER BREATHING AS PER THE BODY'S INSTRUCTIONS

- Sit comfortably.
- Relax.
- Breathe in through the nose.
- Breathe out. Breathe without effort. (If you have difficulty breathing in this manner read footnotes 1 and 2 before proceeding further.)
- Close the mouth.
- Breathe in through the nose. Breathe out through the nose without effort. Continue for a while. (No particular force or effort is necessary.)
- Place you hand over your heart. As you breathe, move your hand up higher, and then down lower to the abdomen.
- Note, as you continue to breathe, where the lungs expand as you breathe in through your nose.

- Once your breathing is relaxed, gently pinch off the nose between the thumb, and middle and ring fingers of the right hand, and breath through the mouth.
- Breathe in through the mouth.
- Breathe out. Breathe without effort.
- Continue breathing in and out through the mouth without effort.
- Place your left hand over your heart. As you continue to breathe move your hand up higher, and then lower. Note where your body expands as you breathe in and out through the mouth.
- Continue for a while until you notice where the expanding and contracting take place. (No force or effort is necessary.)

Depending on whether one breathes through the nose or the mouth the air goes to different locations in the lungs.[1] Once you become aware of this then proceed *to the italicized question below.* If you don't notice a difference then continue the exercise for a few more minutes breathing a bit more deeply, and focusing on the expansion of the lungs. Or return to the beginning of the exercise and breathe more deeply as you follow these steps a second time. (This exercise is important to the reversal of aging as well as to subsequent parts of the course: don't give up unless there is discomfort. If the exercise tires you or there is discomfort then read the footnotes. If necessary take a rest, or even proceed to Session 2 and come back to Session 1 later.)

Note: If you are a Type A personality and have rushed ahead to discover how to breathe properly please return to this exercise and determine for yourself how your body works. Very soon I will report what 99 out of 100 people experience—but do figure it out for yourself.

Breathing through the mouth results in the air going to the upper lungs. Unless you have been trained to breathe diaphragmatically through the mouth (possibly as singer, or as a competitive swimmer) breathing through the mouth results in air filling the upper lungs. When breathing through the mouth naturally—without effort or conscious control –the upper lungs fill with air. Very little air, if any, enters the lower lungs.

THE KEY UNDERSTANDING OF THIS EXERCISE

Where does the air go when you breathe through your nose? Answer: into the lower lungs. Effortlessly and easily, and naturally we could say, the air goes to the lower lungs which supply most of the oxygen to the brain.

BREATHING DURING THE FIGHT OR FLIGHT RESPONSE

The air taken in through the mouth fills the upper lungs. Why? Suppose a nearby car backfires. Our response is the familiar 'fight or flight' response. One gulps air through the mouth and the air enters into the upper lungs but not the lower lungs. Why? Because the upper lungs supply oxygen to the muscles. Whatever has startled us,— a saber toothed tiger or an approaching steam roller—may likely require the use our muscles to respond. Why are we built this way? There are various answers: God built us this way; Nature created us this way; or, early humans who didn't gulp air into their upper lungs to fuel the muscles were eaten by saber tooth tigers, and were subsequently weeded out of the gene pool. For those of us alive today a startle response automatically stimulates us to breathe in air through the mouth into the upper lungs to fuel the muscles with oxygen. (Is this rocket science? Is this esoteric—new age, twilight zone stuff? Not at all—it's simply basic human physiology.)

Notice also how great athletes breathe. Are they performing with their mouths hanging open gulping great gulps of air? No: primarily they use the nose to breathe. Observe also the not so great athletes: the boxer who is defeated; the hockey player who has missed the pass; the gymnast who is struggling. How do they breathe? Most often they breathe through the mouth.

Consider also that hyperventilation is the continuous, rapid, prolonged breathing using primarily the upper lungs to oxygenate the muscles. But often the brain is insufficiently oxygenated and fainting may occur.

EFFECTIVE BREATHING

Breathing through the nose makes use of the lower lungs which results in the intake of more oxygen with less effort. Breathing through the nose makes good sense. Indeed what would be the sense in not using the breathing capacity of the lower lungs? [2]

THE ADVANTAGE OF EXHALING THROUGH THE NOSE

Whether we make use the lower lungs while breathing or not, the body deposits wastes there to be excreted.

This debris must be cleaned out. An added advantage to exhaling through the nose (that we will presently verify) is that air is removed from the lower lungs. I don't know of any research studies on this subject but Ayurveda, 5000 years old, tells us that breathing through the nose cleans the lower lungs.

THE NOSE IS FOR BREATHING

Breathing in through the nose warms and filters the air, and as we have experienced fills the lower lungs with the oxygen needed to fuel the brain. Breathing out through the nose cleans the lower lungs and stretches and tones the muscles around the lower lungs. It seems clear from our experience in this first session that in most cases the nose is preferable over the mouth for effective breathing. [3]

THE BODY HAS INTELLIGENCE

Central to *The Aging Reversal Course* is the idea that by 'listening' to our inner intelligence we can determine how to best give the body the support it requires. At any time since birth we might have noticed that when we breathe through the nose the lower lungs fill with air. This is an excellent example of our body's built in instruction manual. Might there be numbers of other messages within the body waiting to be rediscovered? There are! We only need to focus on the body and be open to these messages to 'hear' them.

While many people breathe properly, many others do not. Prior to the hoards of diet gurus and stacks of research papers how did bygone generations learn to breathe or what to eat? They paid attention to the wants and needs of their body. People who didn't pay attention to this information struggled to survive and were eliminated from the gene pool.

I'm not suggesting that we give up on well researched science. I'm suggesting we add to our scientific knowledge the instructions of our body. Finding these built in instructions is what **The Aging Reversal Course** is about: cues for proper oxygenation, hydration, assimilation, daily routine, euphoria producing exercise. The body has wisdom regarding all areas of Life. We only need to listen and the body will tell us what it wants and needs.

FURTHERING THE EXPERIMENT

By focusing on the outbreath let's expand our understanding of proper breathing. Gently pinching the nose closed as before (through the use of the thumb, and the index and ring finger) and breathe in and out through the mouth for a while.

- Notice that the air is not completely emptied from the lower lungs.
- Make an effort (be easy with yourself) to empty the lungs by breathing out through the mouth.
- Can you completely empty the lower lungs while breathing through the mouth?
- Even while breathing diaphragmatically through the mouth it is extremely difficult, if not impossible, to fully empty the lungs. (How inefficient (and unnatural) to breathe using only the upper lungs.)

- Now breathe in and out through the nose. It should be easy to fill and empty the lower lungs.

For most people, in most situations, breathing through the nose is most efficient, and results in vitality and vigor. Practice this style of breathing and enjoy the difference it makes to your well being once you have incorporated it into your life.

CLEANING THE LOWER LUNGS

(Perform this exercise either alone or in the company of understanding friends.)

- Sit comfortably in a well ventilated room, or outside in fresh air.
- Breathe in and out through the nose. (You can do this exercise most any time of day: during a walk, working in the garden, first thing in the morning. But don't practicing this (or any breathing exercise) when driving, using tools, or doing anything potentially dangerous.)
- After breathing comfortably through the nose gently increase the force of the outbreath—but do not stain.
- Gradually exhale more vigorously until you make a sound much like the one Darth Vader makes as he exhales. The sound is similar to the roar of a crowd at a sporting event.

As a final caution: don't strain. If you find that this breathing exercise takes energy or is stressful then practice it for only a few breaths during your first attempts until you get used to it. [4]

A PERSONAL COMMENT

I spent many decades disregarding this wealth of information but as a word of encouragement I did resumed proper breathing at the age of 45. If you are now beginning to again breathe properly please accept my sincere congratulations. And congratulations to those of you who had the good sense to pay attention to the prodding of your physiology and benefit from proper breathing throughout your entire life.

Now, after having explained all of the above, I am nonetheless sure that somewhere among the great multiplicity of human beings there exists a hale octogenarian who breathes solely through the mouth. Regardless of how healthy this person may be, my guess is that they would have been even healthier had they breathed through their nose.

ATTENTION HEALS

EXERCISE

This exercise provides opportunity to experience the phenomenon that our *attention has the ability to enliven what we focus upon*. Even if you don't become aware of a difference in the quality of your breathing with your attention focused on it nevertheless relax and enjoy whatever you do experience. As **The Aging Reversal Course** continues to unfold there will be many of opportunities to experientially understand the concept that our attention heals.

Practice a set of Darth Vader breathing once a day keeping your focus easily on the breathing.

In addition, at another time, allow this type of breathing to happen naturally with your attention focused on whatever safe task you are performing—for example weeding the garden.

When your attention is focused on the breathing do you notice a sense of enlivenment? (In **Session 3: Our Body as an Ally** and in **Session 18: Quantum Mechanics and Human Physiology** we will discuss further the concept that our attention enlivens what we focus on.)

SESSION WRAP-UP

FOCUS FOR THE WEEK
- Conscious breathing.
- Breathing through the nose.
- At least once a day, preferably in the clean predawn air, focus your attention *easily* on Darth Vader Breathing—particularly the out breath.

EDITORIAL RANT
At an early presentation of **The Aging Reversal Course** regarding breathing one of the participants told me he had read research from a prestigious university indicating that the most effective way to exhale was through the mouth. I have a great deal of respect for science—if I wanted to live in a country bereft of it there are many such hellholes scattered about the planet. But science has made any number of mistakes and we often view it through our cultural filters. The research on red wine is an example. There is research that indicates the moderate consumption of red wine results in fewer cardiovascular problems (I occasionally enjoy a glass of red wine.)—and it appears to be pretty good research. But there is other research—scrutinized under me-

ta-analysis [5]—indicating that any amount of alcohol consumption increases the risk of cancer. The cardio benefits have been widely touted: the second set of info is seldom mentioned. The research from the prestigious university is somehow wrong. The body, if listened to, shows us quite clearly that breathing out through the nose in more effective in removing air form the lower lungs than trying to do this by breathing out through the mouth.

AGING REVERSAL

- The nose is for breathing.
- Effective breathing, in most instances, is accomplished best by breathing in and out through the nose.
- Our body has information about how to breathe efficiently.
- The body has built in instructions.
- Our body has intelligence.
- There are numerous messages within our body waiting to be rediscovered.
- Throughout the ages human beings have lived satisfying lives on the basis of recognizing the intelligence of their body.
- The practice of listening to the body needs to be reintroduced into our culture.

FURTHER READING

Though the reader is encouraged to focus on ***The Aging Reversal Course*** you wish to search out a particular interest. If so check the ***Readings and Websites*** at the end of the course.

FURTHER WRITING

Explore the idea that we create physiology through our thoughts. (Covered in *Session 5: Creating Physiology/ Creating Balance*.)

Recall and describe a time when you felt fully oxygenated. A time when you were so full of Life that you felt you might lift off the ground and float. As you recall and write notice if the feeling is to some degree recreated in your physiology?

> *Note: Although you may create the same effect by just remembering the experience. If you enjoy writing then jump on these opportunities. If an exercise has a double ** it is strongly recommended that you do the writing.*

***

Session 2 outlines proper hydration while *Sessions 3 and 4* present some far reaching and useful ideas.

Session 2
Proper Hydration

THE CHALLENGE OF MAINTAINING PROPER HYDRATION

Western popular culture has recently come to view hydration as key for good health. Eight glasses of water per day is recommended. And lately there has been outrage at the use of plastic to store water, and further concerns regarding the effects of drinking water with high acidity levels. The marketplace offers all kinds of water spinners and hooplacomboobulators which may, or may not, be of use. For most individuals the practice of drinking more water would probably be a good thing but doing so often results in trips to the loo seemingly every other minute.

What to do? What to do?

BOILED WATER

Ayurveda recommends that water be boiled. The reasons for this are several but the main reason is that boiled water is thought to be more easily and quickly assimilated than water that has not been boiled. How could this be verified? I have no idea. You might try drinking boiled water and 'see' if your body is pleased. It may be a 'placebo effect' but when I drink unboiled water I find myself more often running to the loo.

Drink water that has been boiled but drink it at a temperature that suits your preference—hot, warm, or at room temperature. Cold water is not recommended as it requires a good deal of energy to heat it to body temperature.

In addition boiling water helps remove chorine. Water (or anything) that sits in plastic bottles (or plastic pipes) has to be suspect of being less than Life supporting. Find a good source of water and boil it.

SIPPING WATER THROUGHOUT THE DAY

Ayurveda recommends that water be sipped continually throughout the day rather than gulped down glass at a time, though for some constitutions a glass at a time may be just what is needed.

Sipping water prior to, during and after meals may not suit some rare individuals. Listen to what your body is telling you. Your body knows best.

DRINKING DURING MEALS.

Ayurveda contra-recommends large amounts of fluids being taken prior to, during, or right after meals: ie a beer, several cups of coffee, or a glass of ice-water or pop. (See further notes on liquids at mealtimes in **Session 8: Spicing up Your Life.**)

LASSI

The exception to not drinking large amounts of fluids after a meal is the yogurt based drink Lassi. Making your own yogurt is thought to be preferable to commercially prepared yogurt and yogurt is very simple to make. Purchase a yogurt maker (or use the oven on a low heat).

Purchase yogurt starter and follow the instructions which are basically to add the starter to milk and allow the yogurt maker to heat the mixture until the milk turns to yogurt.

To make Lassi mix or blend 1 part yogurt with 1, 2, 3, 4 or 5 parts previously boiled water. Sweeten if desired with sugar or honey or a sweet fruit may be blended into Lassi—mango, peach, cherries etc. Saffron is a nice addition as is toasted cumin powder and salt. Some constitutions may prefer to sip Lassi with the meal but the primary recommendation is to have a glass or two after the main meal of the day. Lassi is not recommended after the evening meal.

BUTTERMILK

Buttermilk either straight up or diluted may be substituted for lassi. It is particularly recommended for constitutions that do not prefer the sour taste of lassi.

CAFFEINE

Caffeinated drinks are contra-indicated for dry constitutions. (Vata Body Types, see **Session 6**) On the other hand the drying effect of caffine is well suited to individuals with an unctuous nature (Kapha constitution). Vaidyas (Ayurvedic Medical Practitioners) talk in terms of a few cups of coffee per week rather than per day. Caffeine, as we have been acculturated to forget, is a drug.

CHAI

A lot of pride is wrapped up in Chai Recipes which are as much prized as the Chili Recipes used in the 'chili cook offs' in the West.

In Ayurveda chai is preferred over coffee or tea as the spices steeped in the chai are thought to buffer the effects of the caffeine. See if this is so for you and experiment to find out what spices best suit your taste.

- While 1 ½ cups of previously boiled water is coming to a boil add whole cloves, cardamom pods and cinnamon bark.
- Other spices may be added such as fennel seeds, fenugreek seeds (bitter), ginger root, licorice root, black pepper, mint and/or saffron (add saffron at the last minute).
- Bring to a boil.
- Add 1 tea bag per 1 ½ cups of water. (Use any type of tea you wish: white, green, decaf. (Is decaf tea natural? Oh these weighty questions.)) Keep the mixture at a low boil.
- When the water has been boiling for a while, or has just begun to gently boil, add 1 ½ cups of milk and bring the mixture for an instant to a gentle boil, and then turn off the heat and let the chai steep. (Boiling the tea is thought to increase the amount of caffine and you may choose to add the tea after the milk has boiled while the chai is steeping.)
- If you must have sugar, first try soaking raisins overnight, or dates (cooling), in the water to be used for the chai.
- Strain, serve and enjoy.
- (Paul's Special Chai: Cloves, cardamom, cinnamon, ginger—skip the tea bag and add instead toasted fennel, coriander and cumin seeds. A

dash of mint on a hot day is a nice touch. (This chai suits me: it may not suit you.))

I have come across individuals who add the chai spices to coffee. This is not a practice from Ayurveda (that I have heard of) but if it tastes good and creates Life supporting effects it may be not only pleasant but useful in balancing the doshas.

FENNEL AND/OR HONEY

For Pitta (the walking furnace constitution) the addition of fennel seeds to a cup or pot of water may provide a pleasing taste and have a cooling effect. (Strain out the seeds) Fennel may improve digestion. Honey is heating and the addition of it may be pleasing for individuals with either a cool or unctuous constitution. (A tablespoon of honey a day is thought to be a great deal of honey. Also, heating honey is thought to turn it to 'poison'. Pasteurized honey is contra-indicated. Cooking with honey is contra-indicated.)

SPICE MIX

Properly spiced water is thought to assimilate more quickly than boiled water. To obtain a spice mix for drinking water that is satisfying to your taste and balancing for your unique constitution consult with a reliable Vaidya who is well trained in pulse diagnosis. (For further information on generic spice mixes for water visit www.mapi.com or www.vaidyamishra.com.)

ACIDIC WATER

Articles too numerous to mention outline the deleterious effects of an over acidic constitution. (See www.

vaidyamishra.com for Vaidya Mishra's article on acidity.) One of the top things you can do to combat acidity is to drink water with a neutral or basic Ph. Purchase some ph paper and check ph level of water you drink. Water with a Basic ph (a ph of 7 or higher is considered to be Life supporting) will be a great help in creating the 7.4, slightly basic level recommended by Ayurveda. Please note that Acidity Level is a complex issue. For example, the stomach, particularly at mealtime, is and needs to be very acidic.

Consider *The Story of the Pancreas* as told to me by a pharmacist.

> *After the stomach has finishing processing a meal with stomach acid the pancreas secretes a basic ph solution into this slurry of digested food prior to it entering the small intestine. Were the pancreas not able to complete this task—for example because of a lack of hydration—two things are likely to happen. The stomach will try to send the food back where it came from which results in acid reflux. Second, the food will pass into the small intestine in a very acidic condition resulting in a 'belly ache'.*

There are no doubt a million reasons for the importance of hydration.

STAYING HYDRATED THROUGHOUT THE NIGHT

Sleeping 7 or 8 or 9 hours through the night (each being normal depending on one's constitution) is a long time to go without water. True, that after adopting the practice of effective breathing from *Session 1* you are now breathing through your nose while sleeping and not waking up with 'cardboard' tongue. And it is also true that the body doesn't require the amount of water during sleeping as it does while active during the day, nonetheless staying hydrated throughout the night is often a challenge.

Ayurveda recommends two things in this regard which we will discuss in more detail in further sessions.

First, soupy dahl or soup (**See Session 8: Cooking**) is recommended for the evening meal. These types of dishes provide better hydration than a meal containing dry foods such as bread and potatoes.

Second, a glass of warm milk is recommended before bed. Somehow a glass of milk is less likely to have one running to the biffy than a glass of water. Warm, pleasantly spiced milk promotes sleep.

Hydration First Thing in the Morning

Before dawn, when you arise, and after cleaning the teeth and scraping the tongue, and so forth, immediately begin sipping, or drinking warm or hot water. If it suits you to work up to 2 or 3 cups first thing in the morning then do so. Add lemon juice to the water, or lime juice if you have a fiery constitution and dislike the taste of sour. Or add your Spice Water spices to the water. Or drink the following tea as per the recipe below.

Why arise before dawn?

When the sun begins to rise, and particularly once it has risen, the body, which has trillions of cells calling out for water, begins to look for hydration. This is particularly true if the body has not remained properly hydrated throughout the night. Where will it get hydration if you don't drink some water? The large intestine. As we know from High School Biology, the large intestine has the ability to extract water from the stool. If the body is not properly hydrated the large intestine will do just that. In addition if your body is not properly hydrated it is very likely that the large intestine will hold on to 'its' supply of water and not 'allow' an early morning bowel movement. (The large intestine, like every other part of the body, has intelligence and will do its duty—in this case by not doing its duty.)

How important is proper hydration to the body's endeavor to repair and keep us youthful? Immense. According to Ayurveda, hydration is absolutely essential for good health. Without it health is impossible.

A YUMMY EARLY MORNING TEA RECIPE (TASTY ANY TIME OF DAY)

Most people, but certainly not all, will enjoy this drink first thing in the morning.

- In the evening place a slice(s) of ginger root, a piece of cinnamon stick or bark, cardamom pods or seeds, pieces of licorice root or licorice powder in a cup (or more) of warm previously boiled water. (See **Reading and Websites** re Vaidya's Mishra's website regarding his DGL product as a substitute for licorice powder if you are concerned regarding the small amount of sugar in the licorice root.)
- Experiment and learn to create an agreeable taste by altering the proportions of the spices in order to concoct a satisfying tea to suit your taste. (This is an important rule for anything you eat or drink: make sure it is suitable to your taste.)

- In the morning warm the tea, strain and enjoy
- Add lemon or lime juice to suit your taste. (Lime juice may be more preferable for some individuals because the secondary taste of lime, after initial digestion, is sweet).

Enjoy.

AROMAS THAT SOOTHE

Note: This session conclude with notes on Aroma Oils and Session 3 concludes with instructions for Warm Oil Massage. Note your preferences for these aroma oils as well as the massage oils as they will later help you determine your Ayurvedic constitution.

Oils with warming and nourishing properties are soothing for individuals who often find themselves cold and dry, and may often daydream of spending a few soothing weeks in Hawaii. Try separately any of the following essential oils in a diffuser. ('Essential' means *essence* or *key ingredient* of the oil as opposed to the more usual meaning of *necessary.*) Clove, Jasmine, Cinnamon, Sandalwood, Clary sage, Lavender, Marjoram.

Cooling and sweet and bitter oils are soothing for individuals who easily overheat and find by October that they are eagerly awaiting the first snow fall. Try Hessop, Lemon, Lemongrass, Mint, Rosewood, Jasmine oils—not mixed, but separately.

Stimulating oils are appropriate for individuals who are cool and moist and find themselves lethargic and/or susceptible to SAD syndrome in the depths of winter. Try Cinnamon, Eucalyptus, Myrrh, Patchouli, Rosemary.

SYNERGY

The Mapi and Mishra websites (see **Reading and Websites**) offers combinations of essential oils designed to pacify Vata, Pitta, and Kapha (which correspond to the three descriptions of the groupings above.) Note that each of these Vata, Pitta and Kapha oils is a synergy of oils designed to create an effect greater than that of its individual components. The reason for combining the component oils is to ameliorate some not so salubrious effects found in individual oils.

The power of synergy is a key concept that is largely employed in Ayurveda and is little understood in the West. (This lack of understanding is found among both pharmaceutical manufacturers as well as new age aroma therapists. Buyer beware!) Some combinations of essential oils may have negative effects and also it is unusual that individual oils will be as effective as properly combined oils.

CREATING BALANCE AT THE QUANTUM MECHANICAL LEVEL THROUGH THE SENSE OF SMELL

Of the three groupings, the first—the 'cold and dry' grouping—may prefer either sesame, almond or apricot oil on the skin. Lavender *or* Marjoram may be mixed with one of these oils and applied to the skin.

For those of us with 'the walking furnace constitution' Lemon *or* Chamomile may be added to Sesame (heating), almond or Coconut oil.

For those with a more mellow nature Eucalyptus *or* Rosemary maybe added to Sesame or Olive oil.

NOTES ON MASSAGE OILS

Sesame oil has a heating quality, but is thought to be the best oil for opening, penetrating and cleaning the pores. Open sesame!

Coconut oil is the most cooling of the oils. Ghee (clarified butter See **Appendix C**) is cooling but is more often used in cooking than on the skin.

Organic oils are recommended as toxins are often oil soluble.

SESSION WRAP-UP

Focus for the Week

Focus your attention on the water you drink: the taste, temperature, texture and the sound and sight of the water. Feel it in your mouth and throat and stomach. Enjoy. You are not fueling the car; instead through drinking you are giving yourself the gift of Life.

Editorial Rant

Note please that **Session 1** deals with Oxygenation and **Session 2** deals with Hydration. Without proper oxygenation and proper hydration any attempt to implement the progressively more complex aspects of **The Aging Reversal Course** will be a challenge. Find a way to give your body the oxygen and water it so dearly needs to do the job it needs to do. If you need a few weeks to focus on these aspects of physiology then do so. I strongly recommend that you have some measure of success with breathing and hydration before you charge ahead with the remainder of the course and possibly become overloaded with things to do. Make proper breathing and hydration and automatic part of your life.

Aging Reversal

- Ample hydration is essential for the body to perform the trillions of functions required for good health. The body is mostly made up of water.
- A well hydrated physiology will function better and last longer than a dried out physiology.
- Staying hydrated throughout the night is absolutely essential for good health, and aging reversal.
- Inadequate hydration leads to premature aging.
- 'Life filled' ph basic water is preferable to acidic water.

Further Reading

Check the www.mapi.com and www.vaidyamishra.com websites for generic spice mixes for drinking water.

Further Writing

Recall and discuss the best water you ever drank.

***

Let's move on to **Session 3** and consider some idea we have touched upon but not fully discussed.

Session 3
Understanding our Body as an Ally

This session elaborates on five key concepts and concludes with instructions for warm oil massage.

CONCEPT 1: THROUGH SELF-INTEREST THE BODY HEALS AND PROTECTS ITSELF

Consider a person who is terminally ill. They wish to pass on and shortly after making this wish they die. What will their body have been doing from the time of the wish and right up until death? Whatever part of the body is functioning will do what it has done since birth: it will work to heal itself. Even when a person wishes to die, even if much of the body's ability for healing has been lost, the body will work diligently to heal itself until the moment Life leaves.

Further regarding the body's self interest: Do we have to tell the body: 'heal my scrapped knee,—Or 'here comes a flu bug!' protect me? No, the body has 'self interest' and we don't need to tell it anything as the body is extremely interested in staying alive. And as long as the body is alive it wants to heal. It tells us to respond if our well being is threatened. For example if we become aware of an approaching steam roller we don't passively stand about thinking, 'Here comes the steam roller. My goodness the steam roller is getting close. Ouch, that is one heavy steamroller—arhhh.' It is unlikely we think at all when threatened. The body has the 'fight or flight' mechanism: we react 'automatically' without any thought.

In the same automatic fashion the body deals with a flu bug or anything that is a threat to normalcy. Through self interest the body heals and protects itself.

CONCEPT 2: THE BODY TELLS US WHAT IT WANTS AND NEEDS

If the body wants a bag of chips every 4 hours is this the work of the 'devil'? No the craving is a message telling us of a need. So do we gobble down a bag of chips? No, our job is to find a way to satisfy this need in a Life supporting manner.

I think it is fair to say, that Westerners (who I am one of), generally believe that the same body that performs trillions of functions per second to keep us healthy is somehow the enemy. There is some apparent basis for this belief when body appears to be destroying itself through disease, but the body primarily wants to stay alive and will tell us what it wants and needs in order to function properly. (See *Session 11: Life*)

CONCEPT 3: THE BODY IS CONTINUALLY CLEANING ITSELF

The body has an amazing capacity for constantly cleaning itself through the proper functioning of the immune, respiratory and excretory systems. Think of dust that gets in an eye; the toxins consumed with our food; the grit breathed in with the air.

We may make a choice as to how to breathe but we have little conscious input into our internal workings. A properly functioning liver, in addition to removing impurities from the blood, also cleans and rebuilds itself automatically. To try to control the functioning of this incredibly complex organ is ludicrous.

This is not to say we can't support the body in its endeavor to clean. Ayurveda has books full of numerous protocols to clean the body and the various organs. For example Vedic exercise, and Yoga Postures (as well as Tai Chi) are designed to strengthen and clean the internal organs. *(Session 10: Vedic Exercise).* And certainly our thoughts, and consciousness, play a large role in our well being. *(Session 18: Quantum Mechanics and Human Physiology).* But the body is well designed to clean itself. We need to give it what it requires (in a Life supporting fashion) and let it do what it so well able to do.

CONCEPT 4: ATTENTION ENLIVENS THAT WHICH WE FOCUS UPON: OUR ATTENTION HEALS

From an Ayurvedic perspective, pain functions to focus our attention on physical **and emotional damage** in order to prompt and assist the body to heal. Our attention, though sometimes painful is part of the process.

(The Darth Vader breathing from **Session 1** is a good opportunity to experience the ability to enliven physiology—in this case enlivening our breathing and subsequently our entire physiology. Focus on your breathing during this deep breathing exercise.)

Our discussions in **Session 10** regarding Yoga Asanas, Suyra Namaskar, Tai Chi, and Vedic exercise will show how these 'exercises' are each designed to draw attention to key areas of the body for the purpose of enlivening the systems of our physiology connected to these areas. This concept that attention heals and enlivens is an extremely important concept in our endeavor to create well being and I encourage you to put your attention on this powerful idea.

CONCEPT 5: THE BODY SEEKS TO MAINTAIN BALANCE

One of the most far reaching concepts of Ayurveda is its understanding of each individual's unique need for balance—a conception that is remarkably in sync with the conceptions of Quantum Mechanics. (*See **Session 18***) Ayurveda posits that there are three first elements of 'matter': **Vata**, which governs movement; **Pitta**, which governs heat and metabolism; and **Kapha** which governs structure and fluidity. Each of us has a unique proportions and amounts of these elements. Creating balance and health is simple: all experience—sensory, emotional, spiritual and intellectual—may be used to regain balance and create dynamic health. (See *Sessions 5 and 6)* Imbalance is understood to be the basis for sickness and aging.

OUR ROLE IN SUPPORTING THE BODY

These five initial concepts are proverbial snowflakes on the tip of the proverbial iceberg that is Ayurveda. What may be clear from understanding these concepts is that the body is our ally though we can't micromanage it. We couldn't attend to 10 functions per second let alone the 6 trillion functions per second the body routinely performs.

The Aging Reversal Course is about how we can give the body what it needs to improve its effectiveness. What can we do right now? Consider what we do when we are injured or sick.

- When seriously hurt we may breathe in far more oxygen. Session 1.
- If we have a cold or flu we rest, drink plenty of fluids, and eat light satisfying foods. Session 2
- As we begin to recover we may do some light exercise or stretching of the damaged part to draw our attention to it. Session 3

In its entirety what we can do to support our physiology is far more detailed and complex than these three simple points but the main message remains the same: we can be proactive in dealing with the stresses of life. We don't have to wait until we are tired to rest, or thirsty to drink, and we can easily give our body the attention and deep rest it so desperately requires. (See **Session 15: Nature's Gift for Dealing with Trauma**)

ABHYANGA: A PLEASANT WARM OIL MASSAGE FOR SUPPORTING THE IMMUNE SYSTEM.

Note: It is not too late to team up with a partner.

The Aging Reversal Course offers much in the way of practical, specific, economical, time-efficient, and enjoyable modalities that may be incorporated into daily routine. Following are instructions for Abhyanga: a warm oil massage that is one of the best things to strengthen your immune system and create balance in your physiology. Also Abhyanga will provide another opportunity to focus your attention and experience your ability to enliven your physiology through this focus.

If your skin is dry and/or you tend to get frazzled and jittery as the day progresses (a sign of Vata Constitution or Vata imbalance) treat yourself to this warm oil massage first thing in the morning. But if your skin is oily to the point that you need two showers a day (Kapha Constitution) then perform the massage without oil. You may find that gloves made of raw silk, or a dry cotton cloth may feel pleasant and that oil is not necessary. ('Feel pleasant'! Yes *The Aging Reversal Course* is about feeling pleasant.)

Light, organic sesame oil is the premier oil recommended by Ayurveda for massage. Of all the oils it is best at opening and cleaning the pores. Sesame oil has a mildly heating effect and may not be suitable to some body types particularly in the summer. If you don't like its smell then heed your body's intelligence and don't use it. Coconut oil may be a better choice for individuals who are constantly hot (a sign of Pitta Constitution or a Pitta imbalance).

- A variety of oils are suitable for massage: almond oil, grape seed oil, olive oil (particularly soothing to sunburned skin).
- High quality, organic oil is recommended as pesticides and other toxicity are often fat soluble. Curing the oil is recommended although the oils will still be effective without curing. *See Appendix A*.

PROCEDURE

- Set a cup or bottle with a small amount of oil in hot water and warm the oil to body temperature (or a bit higher or lower to suit your pleasure).
- Perform the massage in a warm place.

- Cover the floor with a sheet as it is usual to drip some oil during the massage.
- Sip warm water or herbalized tea, and breathe deeply and often during the massage.

In order to test the concept that 'attention enlivens', focus on the area of the body being massaged and at other times during the massage focus elsewhere. (For example look out the window at a tree or flower.) Note whether the differing focus produces different results.

- Begin by applying oil to the head. Massage gently with the palms of the hands.
- Be gentle with the face and most gentle with the neck area between the chin and the collarbones. (Your body will know 'instinctively' to avoid rigorous massaging of this area.)
- The feet, legs, buttocks, hands, arms and shoulders can be fairly vigorously massaged if you wish.
- Stomach and chest should be handled fairly gently.
- The back can be vigorously massaged.
- Use circular motions where it seems applicable, particularly over the joints.
- Clockwise motions are highly recommended. That is to say: if someone were looking at you, your hand would be rotating in a clockwise motion. When massaging the back of the body consider the view as if looking from behind and perform clockwise rotations for this view.
- Use long strokes over the calves, thighs, forearms and arms.

Leave the oil on for as long as is comfortable. The pores of the skin absorb oil and are cleansed by the oil. You will find the skin smoother and you will have a pleasant glow about you. The aroma of sesame oil is pleasant for most people. If it is not pleasant use an alternate oil. Shower with warm water and a high quality liquid soap.

Abhyanga is particularly effective at soothing and balancing Vata dosha. (The doshas are discussed in **Session 6**)

Enjoy the warm oil massage. Don't rush. If your time is constrained then do less massage, but in a leisurely manner.

Note the effects of your attention when focused on the body, and the effects when focused elsewhere. Does your attention enliven the areas massaged?

Additionally there are many uses for sesame oil and these will be discussed in a later session. For example massaging the hands and forearms with oil prior to a painting project will block (to some degree) paint from entering the pores. Or sesame oil may be somewhat effective in protecting a mechanics hands from grease.

SESSION WRAP-UP

Focus for the Week

Abhyanga. Note the experience of your attention enlivening what you attend to. Discuss this in your group. Have you had this experience of 'enlivenment' at other times during your life?

Editorial Rant

How does Ayurveda explain cravings for things known to be destructive to health: heroin, lard, or a pound of sugar?

If the body cries out for a pound of chocolates, or a bag of chips—food that in the long term taxes the physiology—do we blame this craving on the devil, curse the universe for allowing him to temps us and worse yet, curse the universe for encasing us in the weakness of our flesh? No, what we do is to simply figure out what the body really needs. Why would a body, a walking miracle that performs 6 trillion functions per second in order for us to thrive, demand a cup of transfats disguised as potatoes, or for that matter a snort of cocaine? It doesn't really want the transfats or the drugs and considering its usual business of taking care of 'us' (and itself) it must be desperate for something it is lacking. What a novel way to understand cravings! (Dealing with cravings is discussed in later sessions.)

AGING REVERSAL
- In our culture some essential concepts regarding human physiology are pretty much forgotten or in some cases ridiculed.
- The body continually heals, protects and rebuilds itself.
- Attention heals.

FURTHER READING
If you are interested in a quantum leap forward check out physicist John Hagelin's website and look up his comments on the principle of Quantum Mechanics that says that the observer enlivens the observed and visa versa.

FURTHER WRITING
Recall an instance of very rapid healing of a damaged bone or muscle, or a rapid recovery from a sickness. Try to capture the near magic of it and share the experience with your group.

***

Let's move on to **Session 4** which will clear up more of the mythology regarding aging and is also an opportunity to think very specifically about the health you wish to attain.

Session 4
An Alternative Vision of Health and Aging.

AYURVEDA

There are said to be 40 Vedas, Ayurveda being one of them, and they are purported to be, in their entirety, an interrelated blueprint for understanding the workings of the universe. For example Sthapathya Veda is the Vedic understanding of the structure of the universe and everything in it. Dunhra Veda explains all levels of proper defense, from the immune system to how to establish world peace. Gandarva Veda is the complete understanding of sound and music. Ayurveda (Ayur—health, and Veda—knowledge) understands the workings of human physiology cognized and written down thousands of years ago to form the proactive wellness system on which *The Aging Reversal Course* is largely based.

AGING

Determining age by the number of orbits the earth has made around the sun since one's birth seldom provides an accurate measurement of aging. The body is constantly rebuilding itself, and little of it is older than a year. For example none of the cells of the liver are over a year old: this is to say, each cell and therefore the entire liver has been rebuilt anew within the last year. The stomach lining is renewed every day. Skin is constantly being proactively rebuilt to replace skin that is constantly being lost to the wear and tear of living.

The biological age of an individual's body is seldom equivalent to the chronological age. Indeed some aspects of the physiology might be far more aged while others may be comparatively youthful when compared to the norm. In other words the physiology we describe when we refer to a 60 year old is the physiology of an average of the physiological characteristics of all 60 year olds. Very few 60 year olds have the physiology of the average 60 year old.

The downside of expecting to have the characteristic of an average age once we reach that age is that we often get what we expect. [6] Often we think 'I will soon be 30, or 50, or 70, and then I will experience a state of deterioration like all the other 30 or 50 or 70 year olds'. This is seldom the case as later exercises will demonstrate.

But first, by way of contrast to this notion of age based on an average, consider the following. Years ago a television commercial featured an 80 year old man water-skiing. Not far along in the ad the man slipped out of his skis and continued skiing on his bare feet. Seconds later, he clenched the tow rope in his teeth and continued skiing without the help of his hands. Though this person had been on earth for 80 years how old was he? Surely he didn't exhibit the characteristics of an average 80 year old.

Another person of interest in this regard is a woman who took up acting at the age of 89. She found an agent who secured her a role on the *X Files*. Years later when she was nearly 100 her agent remembered her phoning regularly asking with optimism if any acting roles had been found! What youthfulness.

These two elders, and many others like them, remain young after having been on the planet for a considerable number of decades. Why believe that after 60 years one area of physiology is necessarily going to fall apart, and at 70 another faculty will be lost, and at 80 something else will disintegrate?

Hold on to your optimism: it is a very healthy approach to life.

HEALTH

Ayurveda posits that health is not just the absence of disease.

(Webster's Dictionary) Health is the general condition of the body or mind with reference to soundness and vigor.

(A definition that works for me.) Health is a condition of vigor and ebullience supported by the optimal functioning of the physiology.

Your own definition of health need not be perfect but it is important that you begin to choose words, which will shape your thoughts (as words often do) to describe the health you seek.

If our thinking is not promoting a long healthy life let's get headed where we want to end up.

> 'If we don't change directions we are likely to find ourselves exactly where we are headed.'
> A Chinese saying.

***

EXERCISE 1

*It is important that you write a definition of health. Get a notebook. Put your name and the date on it. Title the book as you wish. **My Health; Bob Regains his Youth; Bill loses his love handles, I R Healthy,** or whatever you choose to entitle this record of your progress.*

Write on the first page beginning with the words: 'Health to me is…' Describe the health you want for yourself. Take two minutes to do this. It is okay if it is not perfect. You can revise it later. But for now write down some thoughts so as to establish in your consciousness what you are looking for in terms of health. Do this. It is important in your journey to create aging reversal.

***

YOUTHFULNESS

Consider the following characteristics of youthfulness:

- Good appetite
- Good digestion
- Good eyesight
- Ability of the eyes to quickly adjust to low levels of light.
- Good hearing
- Acute functioning of the *senses*.

- Memory.
- Mental quickness.
- Cognitive flexibility.
- Learning ability.
- Organizational ability.
- Good sleep.
- Strength; flexibility.
- Good gums and teeth.

- Ability to heal quickly.
- Quick recovery from shock.
- Tolerance for heat and cold, and stress in general.
- Vim, vigor vitality and spiritedness.

Wow, it would be great to have all of the above. Children often do. Often regardless of how they strain themselves they emerge pink and shining, full of vigor, ready to charge headlong into activity after a night of sleep. It seems as though youthfulness might be a substance allotted at birth: a fixed quantity of something we burn up as the years pass. At 20, 30, 40, 50 years of age there is noticeably less of it and one may feel that youth has been consumed: appetite is diminished; hearing is less acute; mental ability has slowed; cold bothers us, and for that matter so do heat, and rain. In Ayurvedic thought there is such a substance of youthfulness, called Ojas. The good news is that our body craves Ojas and constantly directs us (loudly and clearly) to live in a manner to facilitate the creation of this marvelous substance.

- A key part of aging is the wanton destruction of Ojas.
- Another key part of the aging process is our failure to help the body create additional Ojas.

One of the primary focuses of **The Aging Reversal Course** is to show each individual how to design a way of living that will satisfy their unique constitution and thereby promote the production of Ojas. Proper breathing, ample water, warm oil massage, spice tea, waking up early, an early morning bowel movement, pleasant exercise: all these and much more are crucial to producing Ojas.

Some translations of the ancient texts regarding Ojas claim that there are only 8 drops of Ojas in the physiology. A yogi listening to a reading of the text corrected the translation saying that there are 8 types of Ojas and altogether Ojas amounts in size to about a handful, primarily located in and near the heart but infused throughout the body. Ojas is the byproduct of proper digestion and proper lifestyle both of which are easily and pleasantly attainable. The notion that Ojas is available in a fixed amount that continuously depletes over the course of life is as erroneous as our western notion that youthfulness is akin to car fuel—something to be consumed never to be had again..

***

EXERCISE 2

Write in your notebook a description of a time that you felt particularly exuberant and youthful. The purpose of this exercise is to establish clearly in your consciousness what you mean by youthfulness. This is a good time to be connected with a group or partner. *Remember a euphoric time: when you ran like the wind, or when you rocked in a rocking chair and felt as though you were going to float up to the clouds.*

Further use of this exercise will be discussed in **Session 5: Creating Physiology**. Our thoughts create our physiology. Enjoy the memory as well as the writing of it.

***

WHY WE AGE

According to Ayurveda, the primary reason for aging is that the cells lose their memory of how to rebuild themselves properly. Cancer is an extreme example of this loss of intelligence. The solution to cancer, and aging, and any disease, from an Ayurvedic Perspective is to know and implement the means of re-enlivening the intelligence of the cells in order that before cancer is established they remember how to recreate themselves properly. **The Aging Reversal Course** is about how to recover our inner intelligence that directs the proper rebuilding of our physiology.

DETERMINING BIOLOGICAL AGE

Determine your biological age so that at the end of the course, and every six months after, you will be able to see your progress.

1) Have your hearing tested. Most hearing centers will test your hearing. Ask them to give you an average age for your hearing and compare that to your chronological age.

2) Have a complete physical, paying particular attention to recording information regarding cholesterol and cardiovascular efficiency. If you don't choose to have the physical then take your blood pressure after a brief walk. Record your blood pressure and heart rate in you note book several times during a week and then again 6 months later.

3) Find a website that offers a good measure of age through a test of mental acuity. Take the test and compare the initial scores with your scores six months later.

Record this data in your IRHealthy notebook. Make the intent that you and your group will retake and discuss these three tests every 6 months after completing **The Aging Reversal Course**.

Years ago a friend studying for a Phd. in Psychology used to repeatedly say, 'There is no knowledge like scientific knowledge.' You want to reverse your aging: be sure that you are having the results you want.

Keep a graph in your notebook to chart your progress.

AVERAGE AGE THROUGHOUT THE GENERAL POPULA-TION.

Average energy levels at every age for the entire population might result in a graph which shows a high point shortly after adolescence and a gradual descent to the low point at death. (See chart.)

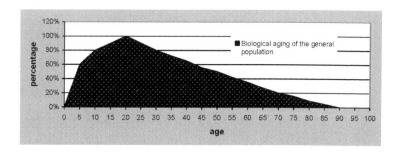

Aging doesn't occur for most individuals in the manner outlined in this graph. I suspect that there have been some ups and downs in the 'optimal functioning' of most people's physiology over the years. Does the graph mirror your aging experience? Does it mirror anyone's? Most likely it does not.

***

EXERCISE 3: CHARTING AGING

Exercise 3 is an opportunity to review your life in terms of the ups and downs of aging. The purpose for charting your aging is twofold. First, it lets you recall times in your life when you were at your most youthful. This memory is a good thing to do for your physiology. (See **Session 5: Creating Physiology**). Secondly, the graph you create will indicate (at least in terms of whatever characteristic you choose to base it on) that you are not sliding down a slippery slope of aging but instead may have had a variety of both setbacks and leaps forward in terms of health and youthfulness. *Can the leaps forward be replicated? Can the setbacks be avoided?* The answer to both questions is a resounding yes.

- Setup a graph in your notebook on the same basis as graph above.
- Sketch a horizontal grid extending across the width of the page.
- And a left hand vertical leg approximately ¼ of the height of the horizontal leg.
- Divide the left hand leg into percentages: 0, 20, 40, 60, 80, and 100. Zero at the bottom.
- Divide the horizontal line into segments of 5 years each, from birth to 100 years of age.

Aging reversal researchers consider an amalgam of factors in determine aging. Usually these include various mental abilities, sensory ability, cardiovascular functioning, reaction to stress (www.tm.org), as well as other aspects of physiology, many of which are listed above in the table **Youthfulness**.

As a first attempt to graph health I suggest you select, as I have, the subjective consideration 'level of energy' or vitality. You may wish to use an alternate indicator of aging: eyesight, hearing, digestion, appetite, or other physiological indices.

First determine an age when your vitality was at its very highest level and mark that high point on your chart as 100%. (It is understood that the level you have chosen isn't an absolutely accurate level of energy but instead your best level of energy thus far in life.)

Review your life and fill in the chart with ups and downs marked as percentages as I have in the chart included below. Footnote the peaks and valleys and describe what was happening in your life to cause these highs and lows.

Though rare, it is possible that you have lived a life of a gradual decline reflected the first graph above. But from my experience most individual's graphs will show peaks and valleys which is a much more accurate portrayal of normal aging.

***

MY YOUTHFULNESS CHART

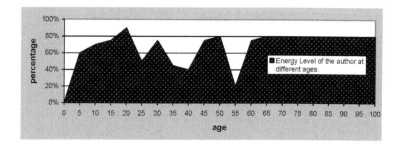

In my late 20's I was in a stressful and unsuitable, sedentary job. My body generally ached. I slept a lot, went to a chiropractor every week, and was generally lacking energy.

By the age of 30, still doing the same work, I was involved in exercise and sports. I had begun dabbling in real estate and building homes as a sideline from my regular work. My energy and self esteem spiked. I had nearly the vim I had when I was 22 when I worked on oilrigs on the Gulf of Mexico. I had largely recovered my vitality.

By my late 30's, through overwork, I had let myself slide into disrepair.

During my mid-40s I was fortunate to be able to treat myself yearly to several weeks of Panchakarma treatments. [7]

In my early 50's my well being spiked resulting from four months in an ashram/health spa that offered PK. I 'worked' nearly stressless five hour days during those wonderful months, eating fabulous food. At the end of the working day a group of us would retire to the hot tub and then the swimming pool prior to evening meditation. More recreation after the evening meal: skating, tobogganing, walking in the forest, or singing lessons. I again regained my vigor. At the end of my stay I had an eight day PK session. I came out of the ashram looking and feeling 20 years younger.

Later in my 50's after 5 years of the rough living that goes with high pressure management consulting work I let myself become sick to the point of dying. I was certain I was old man never to be young again. I convinced myself that even if I did survive, my youth and strength were permanently gone. Somehow I summoned the energy to pull together all that I knew about Ayurveda and built a daily routine that including rest, fun, diet and a exercise program (fortunately based on the Life supporting principles of Vedic exercise) in order to salvage what I could of my life. Today at the age of nearly 64, with a firm promise never to overwork again, I am in many respects as healthy and as vigorous as I have ever been.

COMMENTS REGARDING YOUR YOUTHFULNESS CHART

Though we will make use of your findings later in the course the primary purpose of this exercise is for you to be aware that at times in your life you both lost, and then to some degree regained, your youthfulness. We need to be clear about the way aging happens. **Aging is not a slippery slope of diminishing strength and diminishing youthfulness, it is a fluid and manageable process with ups and downs. We need to focus on the upswings of youthfulness.**

Note the peaks and valleys of your chart. Describe what took place. What caused the aging? You may have lost a loved one or faced a major health challenge. You may have regained your vigor through counseling, volunteer work, and/or the support of your church or spiritual group. How did you reverse the aging? Human physiology is capable of amazing feats of repair and if the physiology of one person has regained youthfulness then potentially any person has the capacity to regain youthfulness. The body desperately wants to be young. You have likely recovered youthfulness in the past and you can recover it again, particularly through *The Aging Reversal Course,* even more profoundly today.

SESSION WRAP-UP

FOCUS FOR THE WEEK

Create the graph and review the ups and downs of aging throughout your life. What did you introduce into your life to help you recover?

If you are enjoying Abhyanga and still find that you are dry, or still don't sleep well at night, massage the feet and hands with a suitable oil prior to sleep.

Editorial Rant

What a brainwash it is to believe that after having been on the planet for 60 orbits around the sun a person will be "60 years old." Some of us will be in the shape of an average 40 year old; some of us will be '80'; and some of us will be dead. Some will have some systems that function like the average for all 70 year olds, and at the same time have another system that functions like the system of an average 20 year old. What is this need to tag ourselves with an age based on the revolutions of the earth around the sun—particular when the tag provides very little information of use? I have no objection that people know that I have been on the planet 64 years, but I object strongly to most of the conclusions drawn from that information. I don't see that a useful and accurate conclusion can be drawn from it.

Aging Reversal

- There is little evidence to support the idea that the body is a machine that inexorably wears out.
- Youthfulness is not a finite quality that slowly evaporates.
- Within a group of individuals used to make up 'an average age' is a percentage of individual who are far removed from the characteristics of the average.
- Aging has little to do with how many times the earth revolves around the sun.

- Aging is seldom a process without ups and downs.
- Individuals may age and then recover.

FURTHER READING

For quantum leap see Dr. John Hagelin's comments on the immortal nature of sub atomic particles.

FURTHER WRITING

** Recall a time in detail when you were exuberant and youthful. (Two asterisks indicate that this exercise is highly recommended.)

***

Now that you have clearer idea of the physiology you wish to create let's move on to some basic concepts about how to create this ideal physiology, next in **Session 5: Creating Physiology**,

Session 5
Creating Physiology/ Balancing Physiology

BALANCE THROUGH THE SENSES

We constantly re-create our physiology.

Suppose while walking through the woods we come upon a great, long snake coiled and sunning on a rock and suppose we love snakes. "Oh look at his/her lovely, scaly skin. Oh how cute. He is opening his eyes and flicking his tongue. And look he has a lump in him: I bet he has just eaten a mouse. Oh yes, it is still moving." We take a picture and post it on our computer screen. We are in bliss. Or quite possibly, just thinking of the snake fills us with revulsion.

For a person who enjoys snakes, (and these folks do exist) the snake elicits pleasant emotions and thoughts. From the Quantum Mechanical level our thoughts and emotions 'make the leap' to physiology. In the case of the person who love snakes, endorphins (matter resulting from our thoughts) course through the body.

The manner in which we choose to react to life experiences: sensual, emotional, intellectual, spiritual—indeed through any experience human physiology is capable of experiencing—results in physiology. Endorphins (or in the case of a person repulsed by the snake, adrenalin) are created. Physiology has been created from thought and emotion and this new creation interacts with and effects existing physiology.

And our unique filtering and interpretation of experience creates unique physiology. Who makes the decision as to how we react to the snake? God? The stars? No, our reaction is determined by us. The resultant physiology, and the health resulting from all our accumulated experience, is in effect our creation.

When we are ill do we say (and think): 'I'm sick'? Or do we say 'I'm recovering.'? Do we say regarding a backache: 'I have a bad back', or 'I have a good back that I need to continue treat well and manage carefully?' Our thinking effects our physiology.

It may seem harsh that through an innocent thought we create physiology but in fact, it is very good news. This ability allows us to create vibrant health.

GENETICS

What about genetics? If a person chooses to be horrified by the snake, and their genetics include a weak heart, the result might be a heart attack. A different choice might not result in a heart attack. The Zen expression 'Life in is pain; suffering is optional.' suddenly one day upon reflection made sense to me.

Sometimes though, it may seem that we don't have much of a choice. We accidently step on a snake, or we are born in a slum in Mumbai. Nonetheless we still have the choice of how to react. We can fill our physiology full of the chemicals of rage or we can fill our physiology full of the chemicals of joy. [8]

As another example, suppose we have been damaged as a child and years later we rage away at our tormentors. We fill ourselves with the toxic chemicals of rage. Who suffers in this situation? There is no doubt that the injustice happened and the pain of the experience may be very real today. Yet here also we have a choice. We can choose to forgive—not to condone—but to give up on producing the toxic chemicals of rage that are aging us, and to enjoy the chemicals resulting from forgiveness that will permeate our heart and entire physiology.

And certainly we can choose to not consume the box of chocolates, the bottle of tequila or the snort of cocaine. (See **Session 15** regarding dealing with cravings.) We always have a choice. [9]

BEHAVIORAL RASAYANAS: PRESCRIPTIONS FOR LIFE SUPPORTING ACTION.

Ayurveda provides us with direction as to how to act in a manner that promotes balance. As well, practicing these principles of right action resonates within our physiology, and indeed over the years, out of self interest, our physiology has prompted us to act according to these Life supporting dicta. When we contravened these supportive ways of living our body must feel the shock of doing so.

- Avoid anger. Find a way to recognize the first signs of anger and to deal with it by putting the attention on it before it erupts. This means to mitigate—to dissolve or evaporate the anger—not to repress it. There is a time for anger.
- Don't over use the senses. To be discussed in **Session 13**

- Remain calm. Breathe deeply through the nose. **Session 1** Stay cool, i.e. not overly warm.
- Cleanliness of body and environment is important.
- Give. Work not to get money but to give the service you are best suited to give.
- Be respectful.
- Be loving.
- Speak the truth.
- Speak and think well of others.
- Maintain an orderly lifestyle.
- Be guileless. (Do many of these qualities remind you of Mahati Ghandi?)
- Avoid fools and associate with the wise. (Reminiscent of the Desiderata)
- Be positive: be optimistic.
- Follow your cultural traditions—including religious injunctions.
- Focus on spiritual progress.
- Be yourself.
- Listen to The Silence. Learn to experience Silence.
- Respect and care for yourself.

We create physiology every minute of every day. Practicing any of these Rasayanas: respect, optimism, guilelessness, etc, results in physiology. On the other hand disrespectful, pessimistic, and guile also result in physiology. Physiology (my body and your body) encourages Life supporting ways of living because following these principles builds the healthy physiology the body is self interested in having. Physiology discourages contravening these Rasayanas. How do you feel listening to a fool? How do you feel when badmouthing someone? The body is self interested in health: it will tell you when you are destroying your Life force, and it will support you when you are increasing your Life force. Though our best course of action is to listen to the body and act on the basis of its intelligence nonetheless spontaneously introducing these Rasayanas into your life by focusing on each of them one at a time until they become second nature will be good practice until these ways of acting are spontaneous. [10]

BALANCE THROUGH THE SENSE OF TASTE.

For most individuals, most of the time, the sense of taste is the most effect lever for creating balance, health and aging reversal other than through Consciousness (**Session 18**), and practice of the rasayanas listed above. Satisfying our taste requirements is a great key to our well being. Indulging in, or tolerating disagreeable tastes, makes achieving and maintaining balance difficult. (See **Session 6**)

TONGUE MAPPING.

(I hope you are working with a partner who has a sense of humor.)

Ayurveda considers that there are six tastes: sour and salty, sweet and bitter, astringent and pungent. To create balance, all of the six tastes should be satisfied in at least one meal each day. 'Satisfied' will have a different meaning for each individual, and the requirements for being satisfied will likely vary for each individual from day to day. **Session 9: Seasonal and Daily Routines**

***

Taste Mapping Exercise

Set out at least one food from each of the following taste groups:

- **Sour**: plain yogurt, sour cream, lemon or lime, or anything sour.
- **Salty**: Salt, dulse or seaweed.
- **Sweet**: Sugar, honey.
- **Bitter**: Neem, dandelion root, fenugreek, lemon rind, ground coffee.
- **Astringent**: Turmeric (also bitter), alum, pomegranate.
- **Pungent**: Pepper, ginger, cayenne, chili peppers.

In your **I R Healthy** Notebook draw a large U shape to represent the tongue.

Next, rub some of the sour food on the tongue.[11] Note that some tastes register only on a certain area(s) of the tongue. Mark that area(s) on your tongue map. After tasting each taste rinse the mouth and/or clean the tongue with your tongue scraper between tastings. As you rinse the mouth you may notice taste buds on the roof of the mouth or at the back of the mouth. Make note of these also.

In addition make a note of your preference for each taste using a 1 to 10 scale, 10 indicating the greatest preference.

Map each of the six tastes on the U shaped sketch.

***

You now know the tastes you like and those you don't like, and you know where in the mouth the various centers of taste are located. You may have even found some taste buds you didn't know you had and you may have found some areas of taste that you have overlooked for years.

A lot of us grew up eating meat and potatoes and two vegetables because that was what was available. We got in the habit and that diet became, for us, 'normal'. What is truly normal is that all the six tastes and all the taste bud get satisfied. Not using taste buds is much akin to breathing through the mouth and not making use of the lower lungs. What are the lower lungs there for? What are the taste buds for? Did the Creator make a mistake?

SATISFYING THE TASTES

Keeping in mind that your taste requirements vary daily, how will you satisfy all the six tastes, and particularly your preferred tastes?

As you are eating every day anyway I suggest you put your attention on the sense of taste and experiment to eventually find spices and foods that are well suited to your palette. In addition, find a knowledgeable Vaidya and have him/her prescribe a spice mix for cooking as well as a spice mix to add to your drinking water. These mixes are designed specifically for you and are called churnas.

You can purchase generic churnas of good quality organic spices at the websites listed in *Reading and Websites*. You can order churnas called **Vata Churna**, **Pitta Churna** and **Kapha Churna**. Vata churna pacifies Vata dosha, or Vata imbalance; Pitta—Pitta; Kapha—Kapha.

Or you can create your own churnas by trial and error. To begin, adjust this generic mix to suit your taste:
- Mix 1 part turmeric, 1 part cumin, 6 parts coriander and 1 part fennel.
- Along with these spices the tastes of the food and the other spices you normally use in your

meal should provide all 6 tastes in the proportion needed for you to be satisfied. [12]

- If possible grind whole organic seeds, except for turmeric which will be hard to find in a form which lends itself to grinding.
- Initially mix only a small batch of these spices.
- Add these spices into one of the dishes at your main meal.
- The dish you choose—vegetables for example—should have both fat and water in it.
- If you are alone or you are cooking for others who are not interested in new tastes (what a pity), put a half teaspoon of the spice mix in ghee (clarified butter, see **Appendix C**) and heat the mixture until it gives off a pleasant aroma. Then drizzle it on one portion of your meal.
- To alter the spice mix, add in another part turmeric and/or fennel in order that it will be more suitable to your taste. Over time keep adding to the mix until you find it satisfying.
- If you do not like one of the four basic spices then delete it from the mixture. (Never eat something that is not pleasing.)
- If you have a spice that you have an urge to add to the mix then do so. Ginger, fenugreek, basil, celery seed, and cinnamon might be of interest.

Most, but not all individuals, should keep the cumin and coriander at the initial levels of 1 and 6 respectively unless you strongly sense that you should adjust them. If so then go to ratios of 1 and 5, and then 1 and 4, etc. [13]

- Minimize the fennel if you don't fancy the taste but keep some in your churna unless it is disagreeable for you. Fennel tones the digestive system but has a cooling effect.
- Turmeric is an anti-oxidant and purifier. When introduced to turmeric most people fall in love with it. If you don't like the taste still include at least some small amount and try to increase the amount gradually, unless you find it entirely disagreeable.

Have fun!

A Generic Vata Churna recipe for satisfy and pacifying Vata constitutions or individuals with Vata imbalance.

In all recipes alter amounts of the ingredients to suit your taste.

In all recipes begin by including larger amounts of the first spice and progressively lesser amounts for each of the following spices.

Generic Vata Churna.
- Cumin, ginger, fenugreek, turmeric, brown sugar, salt, asafetida (hing).

Generic Pitta Churna.
- Coriander, fennel, cumin, brown sugar, cardamom, ginger, turmeric, cinnamon, salt.

Generic Kapha Churna.
- Ginger, pepper, coriander, brown sugar, turmeric, salt, cinnamon.

Experiment! Add additional spices. Make mealtimes a symphony of taste.

TASTE AS A KEY TO UNDERSTANDING CONSTITUTION.

Ayurveda posits that on a quantum mechanical level, at the level of first 'matter', far below electrons, far below quarks, close to the basis of all creation, is the beginning of three primordial 'elements':

Vata: responsible for movement, characterized by cold and dry.

Pitta: responsible for heat and metabolism, characterized by hot and moist.

Kapha: responsible for structure and fluidity, characterized by cool and moist. [14]

According to Ayurveda, each of us (and indeed everything 'physical' in the universe) is made up of a combination of these first manifested elements, but set up in a unique fashion and in unique proportions which results in our individual physiology. [15]

In Ayurveda taste is used to pacify and balance Vata, Pitta and Kapha.

- Salty and Sour tastes pacify **Vata**.
- Sweet and Bitter pacify **Pitta.**
- Astringent and pungent pacify **Kapha.**

If, in your taste mapping, you preferred salty and sour tastes you may have a preponderance of Vata in your make up (you are cold, dry, slight of build, quick and lively) or though your original constitution is Pitta or Kapha you have a Vata imbalance that your body is attempting to rectify through these tastes.

Sweet and bitter indicate Pitta constitution or imbalance.

Astringent and pungent indicate Kapha.

During at least one meal a day (preferably at the noon meal and indeed each meal if possible) all six tastes should be included in proportions that are pleasing and suitable to what the physiology requires. Not the tastes the cook decides. Not the tastes some diet guru decides. Not a meal based on mineral and amino acids requirements but a meal designed for, and by, your taste buds.

If you wish to add vitamins and so forth to your meals go right ahead. Note that people who lived prior to 100 years ago, and people living today in 'primitive' cultures where longevity is usual have not heard of a vitamin much less an amino acid. Why did they thrive? First, they choose to live in a place that provided them with their nutritional needs. Second, they had the good sense to eat on the basis of their body's intelligence: that is, **they ate what pleased their sense of taste, and they ate what made them feel alive and energetic**. It is unlikely that one of these centenarians would ever be found holding their nose gagging as they tried to choke down some goop they had whipped up in a blender. They ate food.

Individuals whose nutritional needs were satisfied remained in the lands that provided what they needed, and they thrived. Those whose needs were not met moved on, or died off. For example the Inuit living in the Arctic thriving on whale blubber, or the indiginous people in the Andes Mountains living on spuds and minerals from the rocks are excellent examples of physiology that was able to thrive on what the environment provided. Those who could not survive on these diets died out and their genetics were quickly removed from the gene pool.

TASTES THAT AGGRAVATE THE DOSHAS

- Sweet, Sour and Salty aggravate **Kapha**. Kaphas please begin gradually refraining from sugar and the overuse of salt. A wee bit of honey once or twice per day may be okay.
- Pungent, Bitter and Astringent (dry) aggravate **Vata**. (Vatas please stay off the coffee. You are not the pretty sight you think you are when bouncing around on numerous cups of caffine.) The spice turmeric is astringent and has a drying effect and though a bit of it is good, a lot may be aggravating.
- Pungent, sour and Salty aggravate **Pitta**. When I was a boy, I would gather with my friends and looking on in anticipation we would beg my Dad to eat a pickle so we could watch the sweat 'pop out' on his forehead. In slow motion, within a few seconds after biting into the pickle, beads of sweat would ooze out on dad's forehead. Sour is most aggravating to **Pitta**.

If you find any of the above tastes aggravating, then this is another clue to your constitution. While it may be the case that through habit one has learned to like an unsuitable taste (a Kapha who prefers sweets) it is also likely that you have a sizeable Kapha component if the tastes sweet, sour and salty are your least favorite tastes, or tastes you find aggravating.

The doshas may be aggravated in any of a gazillion ways other that poor food choices. For Vata a lack of routine, skipping meals and sleeping at irregular times, and a cluttered house or work place will do the job. For Pitta, heat, mental strain and overwork. For Kapha, lack of stimulation, sugar, fat, sleeping in, and laying about. Food is a great key for balancing the doshas but when misused it results in imbalance.

Meat

Meat often has each of the six tastes and is though it is usually considered sweet when first eaten it often produces a sour effect as it is digested. See *Session 11: Life*.

Satisfying Tastes Through the Use of Spices.

Over the millennia tastes have been satisfied most pleasantly by including the judicious use of spices in cooking. Spices can easily satisfy all the six tastes. In addition spices carry nutrients readily to the cells. Treat yourself at every meal. Make every mouthful rapturous. Make the meal a gift: an offering to you—HUGELY IMPORTANT AND DESERVING YOU!

What spices do you like? The sweet spices: cinnamon, nutmeg, saffron etc? How about turmeric, basil or dill? How difficult would it be to include into your diet each day spices that thrill your taste buds? It is an inexpensive, simple, and wonderful thing to do for yourself. Even if you eat lunch at work you could bring a packet of dill or a few strands of saffron to sprinkle on your food. But make changes slowly. Don't get overwhelmed.

What other spices do you like? Salt and Pepper. Fenugreek? (It smells and tastes like butterscotch.) Mustard seeds, cloves, cilantro? A whole symphony of taste awaits you. Smell the spices. Does the smell please you? Try it out. Never mind what Sister Mary Mary Mary of the <u>Blessed Order of the Sour, Bitter, Astringent Convent of No Spices and No Fun Allowed in Our Convent</u>, taught you.

The savory smells of spices, grains and veggies cooked in ghee is coming from my kitchen and preparing my physiology for lunch. I hope the little rant above doesn't lessen my enjoyment of it.

SESSION WRAP-UP

FOCUS OF THE WEEK

- Continue to further understand your taste requirements and find ways to satisfy them.
- Note the aromas you prefer and focus on the delightful variety of aromas in your environment.
- Incorporate the Behavioral Rasanyas into your life.

EDITORIAL RANT

No matter how severe your programming regarding sensuality dig into the spices. Honest, it is okay to enjoy.

I grew up eating meals of meat and potatoes, and two vegetables. (Usually one of them was carrots.) Once in a while there was fish; macaroni and cheese; and on occasion a wildly exotic dish we called Spanish Rice. (Rice baked with tomato sauce with sliced hot dogs and topped with a crust of cheddar cheese.) Mom was a great cook but that was the food we had. Spices were salt and pepper; cloves baked in roast ham; and cinnamon on French toast. Mom told us that cinnamon was tree bark and that put most of us off cinnamon for a while.

AGING REVERSAL

- Food is an offering. Sensuality is important. Stretch your taste boundaries.
- We create our physiology through our choices.

- Our body's intelligence has always prompted us to follow Life supporting behavior. This phenomenon is an excellent example of Natural Law at work.
- Balance on the grosser levels (for example the body's acidity level) is important. Far more important is balance on the subtler levels of Vata, Pitta and Kapha.
- Taste, and all the senses as well as our thoughts, emotions, surroundings may be used to balance our physiology.

FURTHER READING

Nearly every book on Ayurveda has a chapter on creating balance through taste.

FURTHER WRITING

Describe a time when you felt energized after a meal. Describe the meal: not only what you ate but the circumstances surrounding the meal. Who was with you; where you were; time of day; season of year; what had happened earlier in the day.

***

Session 6: Understanding our Uniqueness focuses on gaining insight into our constitution through the use of the best Ayurvedic Body Type questionnaire available.

Session 6
Individuality from an Ayurvedic Perspective

DETERMINING OUR UNIQUENESS

Each individual has a unique physiology with a unique set of requirements in order to maintain balance and health and youthfulness.

Throughout the millennia the majority of humanity has designed diet and lifestyle on an entirely intuitive basis yet an understanding of body type will probably be of use. To provide further insight into your unique body type a questionnaire is provided in *Appendix Q*. (Your preference for aroma oils and massage oils and your taste preferences will have provided a number of initial clues.)

A Caution Regarding the Use of Questionnaires.

Questionnaires seldom account for imbalances which often skew the findings and result in an inaccurate assessment of body type. This concern is dealt with in *Session 7: Cycles of Imbalance* where there will be an opportunity to refine your initial findings by discounting imbalances from your totals.

THE DOSHAS

Ayurveda posits that on a quantum mechanical level, at the level of first 'matter', close to the basis of all creation, there are three primordial doshas ('elements'):

Vata, responsible for movement.

Pitta, responsible for heat and metabolism.

Kapha, responsible for structure and fluidity.

In human physiology Vata predominance is characterized by a cold and dry constitution; Pitta by hot and moist; Kapha by cool and moist. [16]

According to Ayurveda, each of us and indeed everything 'physical' in the universe is made up of these first manifested elements. And while each of us have each of these three elements in our constitution, these **Doshas** are set up within us in a unique fashion and in unique proportions which results in each individual's unique physiology.

Ten Basic Constitutions

For simplicity of discussion Ayurveda divides the over 6 billion unique human constitutions currently on the planet into 10 basic constitutions.

Three of these are commonly referred to as Single Doshic (Single Element) Constitutions. (The word 'single' is not accurate in that everyone has each of the three doshas. It would be more accurate to say 'constitutions dominated by a single element but who wants to say that repeatedly?)

These single doshic constitutions are:

Vata,

Pitta,

Kapha.

There are six Bi-doshic Constitutions (combinations of 2 of the three primary dosha) in which 2 elements are dominant, with the third element seldom if ever dominant or pronounced.

Vata-pitta,

Vata-kapha,

Pitta-vata,

Pitta-kapha,

Kapha-vata,

Kapha-pitta.

The tenth and rarest of the Ayurvedic body types is the Tri-doshic constitution: the *Vata-pitta-kapha* constitution.

A Cursory Description of Single Doshic Constitutions

Vatas are quick and lively: individuals who are dry, sometimes almost seemingly brittle, and cold with dry skin, cracked lips, and fly away hair. Vata's dream is to live in tropics.

A Pitta may stroll about in 20 degrees below zero without a hat and their coat unbuttoned. These individuals like to stay cool in the summer. It is unlikely you will get them to sunbathe. Pittas are often driven, or drivers and their favorite phrase might be "Let's get the job done."

If you are seeking a quick and lively personality seek out a Vata. If you want to get a job organized seek out Pitta, but if you seek stability then choose calm and steady Kapha. Kaphas act and move slowly, usually taking time to 'digest' the situation. As a rule they are slow to get excited. They may have a quality of peace and serenity about them.

Vata is characterized as quick and lively, Pitta as sharp and fiery, and Kapha as ponderers and reliable.

Below is a chart with further characteristics of Vata, Pitta and Kapha. Note that on the basis of percentages there might be 1/3 of the people on earth with a large component of **Vata**, another 2 billion with high **Pitta,** and another 1/3 with high **Kapha**: but keep in mind the phenomenal variety found within the human family.

	VATA	PITTA	KAPHA
Primary Qualities.	Movement.	Heat/Metabolism.	Structure/Fluidity.
Additional Characteristics.	Vivacity, liveliness, quick and sprightly.	Enterprising, Sharp.	Steady, stable, cautious.
Approach to life.	Quick to act.	Competitive.	Slow to take action.
Spiritual inclinations.	Joyous, blissful, ecstatic.	Compassionate, Understanding.	Devoted, devotional.
Signs of Imbalance.	Nervous, anxious, Worried.	Angry, sarcastic, Fanatical.	Depressed, lethargic, Greedy.
Tendencies when imbalanced.	Scattered. Busy, but getting little accomplished.	Domineering, Authoritarian.	Obstructive, stubborn, Childish, maudlin.
Focus in life.	Creators.	Preservers.	Stabilizers or destroyers.
Focus when imbalanced.	Let's change everything.	Let's keep the status quo no matter what.	Let's play Idi Amin.

There are over 6 billion unique constitutions on earth. The table generalizes to provide an initial understanding of Vata, Pitta, and Kapha.

A SECOND CAUTION REGARDING QUESTIONNAIRES.

While it is useful to have an understanding of your body type don't let the conception you come up with from the questionnaire overrule what your body is telling you. Focus on your body's intelligence rather than what a questionnaire and/or textbooks tell you. If a food doesn't taste good don't eat it regardless of what the books say!

IMBALANCES

Your constitution was largely established at the time of conception or certainly by the time of birth. Over the years you may have accumulated imbalances. The two day old child you once were didn't crave a box of chocolates—or bag of chips—or an aged steak. True, as the child grew there were more dietary requirements than milk and pablum. Nonetheless if we refer to the principles of **Session 3**, particularly that the body wants to heal, we may choose to view the source of cravings as arising from a need that has not been met. From an Ayurvedic perspective cravings result from an imbalance of the doshas meaning that the doshas are out of proportion and/or location as per the original constitution. So even if you are beset with an imbalance, continue to work on understanding your unique constitution by developing a better ability to listen to the body and to then become better able to determine what the body requires in order to create balance. [17]

Now proceed to **Appendix Q** and complete the questionnaire as instructed. Once complete, return here and continue reading.

POST QUESTIONNAIRE WORK.

Do the results from the questionnaire seem to accurately describe your constitution? Are you, for example, predominately dry, cold and constantly dreaming of the tropics and your scoring indicates that you have a large Vata component? Or do you eagerly await the snowmobile season and if so Pitta is a better descriptor? Or are you comfortable on the chesterfield leisurely awaiting the next meal—which, in your imagination, you smell and taste.

Does the result of your answers to the questionnaire seem to fit with what you know about your basic nature? For example if your scores indicate a bi-doshic Vata–Kapha then heat is not a problem for you and in fact you love heat. You may have good strength and agility and are able, or were once able, to frolic about all day in the sun.

Do you feel relatively comfortable that the result of the questionnaire is an accurate description of your constitution? If accurate, this understanding will be of use throughout the remainder of the course, and throughout your life. Or are you completely befuddled? If you have some doubts then count yourself one of many. In **Session 7: Cycles of Imbalance** further discussion will lead to understanding Ayurvedic Constitution and there will be an opportunity to review the questionnaire and delete questions that may have skewed the scoring.

Don't worry: be happy!

A CHANGE OF PACE: AN ADDITIONAL BREATHING EXERCISE

If you practice Vedic Exercise, specifically Surya Namaskara, then move on to **Session 7** as you will know this information regarding proper breathing.

Suyra Namaskara (The Sun Salutation, **See Appendix E**) is a highly effective and enjoyable exercise that is again discussed in **Session 10**. I recommend that you find a qualified instructor and learn the exercise with proper guidance. For now, let us first learn, and then consider, what the first 3 postures of the exercise have to tell us about breathing with a view to incorporating this style of breathing into our exercise, work and any other area of life where it may be applicable.

EXERCISE

- *First* posture of the Sun Salutation is to stand (preferably at dawn facing east) with feet together.
- Hold the hands together in Namaste position (as though in prayer).
- Breathe out. Breathe normally.
- *Second* posture: Allow the hands and arms to drop slowly to the sides, and then raise the arms and hands over the head. Don't strain. Arch the back but only if it is easy to do so.
- What is going on with your breathing as you do this? (As you raised your arms the rib cage expands, and then this is a good time to breathe in.)
- *Third* posture: touch the toes. (Easily, do not strain, bend only as far as comfortable.)

- What is going on with the breathing as you do this? (As you begin to bend the rib cage begins to contract and the air is forced out of the lungs. As you continue to bend this is an opportune time to breathe out. By the time you touch the toes (or get as close to them as you are easily able) the lungs should be empty. (Do not lock the knees: keep them slightly bent as you perform this phase of the exercise.)
- Return to the standing position hands over the head in the *first position*. As you do this the rib cage expands and you breathe in.
- Perform Namaste, breathe normally and then lie down and take a brief rest.

Incorporate this style of breathing into your activity. When you reach for something on a high shelf, breathe in. When you bend to pick something up breathe out. Apply this breathing to your exercise program as well as to your work.

SESSION WRAP-UP

FOCUS FOR THE WEEK
- Listen to what your body requires in order to create balance.
- Refine your understanding of your constitution.
- Breathe in when the rib cage is expanded.
- Breathe out as the rib cage begins to contract.

EDITORIAL RANT
We are each blessed with entirely unique physiology. Why the medical profession and the culture can't accept this is beyond my understanding. Normal heart rate is

thought to be 72 beats per minute. What about those of us who's heart rate ranges everywhere else between 30 and 100 bpm.

Obesity is determined by a ratio of girth to height. What about the naturally heavy individuals who can to sink to the bottom of a swimming pool and lie on the bottom like a stone? Are they obese or just naturally heavy?

Our cultural penchant for being 'normal' and meeting an 'average' is most often simply nonsense. 'Normal' is unique for each individual. To believe and practice otherwise is usually destructive.

Aging Reversal

- Each of us is unique.
- The questionnaire results are helpful when added to our intuitive understanding our constitution. To believe the questionnaire and disregard the body's intelligence is in most cases a mistake.
- Considering our body's preferences—particularly for aromas and tastes—is likely more helpful in understanding our body type than the findings of the questionnaire.
- Through focus on our body during the initial postures of the Sun Salute we gather further information from within our body about how to breathe effectively.

Further Reading

Many of the books in the **Reading and Websites** can expand on this session. Lad's book has a great deal of detail regarding physical clues to constitution—fingernail shapes, lips, eyes and the like. Be cautious with this info much in the same way you are cautious with the results of the questionnaire. Trust your intuition.

FURTHER WRITING

Describe someone you know or have met who well fits the descriptions of one of the primary, single doshic constitutions.

***

Next *Session 7: Cycles of Imbalance*

Session 7
Cycles of Imbalance: Further Understanding of Prakriti and Vikriti

---

UNDERSTANDING CONSTITUTION

Prakriti (Pra' kra tee) is the Sanskrit word for constitution or physiological make up—ie one's original constitution. Some individuals understand their Prakriti very quickly, and very well: some not so quickly. I was sure I was Vata. Dry skin, thinning hair, quick to learn—quick to forget, under weight, often worried, etc.

The Vaidya took my pulse and said 'Pitta.'

I replied 'Not Vata?'

'Pitta.'

'Pitta-Vata?'

'Pitta'.

I was sure he was wrong.

Several years and several consultations later (and also because many of the Vata imbalances evaporated) I finally accepted that the real challenge for me was Pitta.

In my case I appeared to be Vata. It is easy to mistake Vikriti for Prakriti: that is to mistake imbalance for constitution. Vikriti is the Sanskrit word for imbalanced physiology.

What to do? What to do?

CYCLES OF IMBALANCE

Consider the main signifiers of Vata, Pitta and Kapha.

Vata: Cold and Dry
Pitta: Hot and Moist
Kapha: Cold and Moist

Suppose one has a predominately Pitta Constitution: that is high metabolism and a preponderance of heat. We have met these people: they walk around with coat open, without a hat in below freezing weather. They love ice cream, and drink ice water with meals. Often they burst into anger over nothing. But once their 'fire has died' they are not able to eat as they once did and may not appear to be Pitta in the least. (Keep in mind there is a great variety in the hundreds of millions of Pitta constitutions living on the planet.)

PITTA-VATA CYCLE OF IMBALANCE

The key characteristic found in Pittas is that they generate huge amounts of heat. What does heat do? It dries. In the Pitta-Vata cycle of imbalance too much heat dries the body resulting in dry skin, dry hair, dry stomach etc, etc. Too much Pitta results in a Vata imbalance. Should we deal with the Vata or the Pitta? Both. But to deal with Vata only, as is so often the approach, is to miss the root of the problem.

VATA-KAPHA CYCLE OF IMBALANCE

One of the key characteristic of Vatas is that they are dry. Dryness may be exacerbated by living in a dry climate or by constant activity and movement, improper routine and rushed meals. Vatas become dry and what, in its wisdom, does the body call out for? What kind of food is craved?

Kaphogenic food: oily, greasy food in order to mitigate the dryness. Eating too much greasy food may pacify Vata but it aggravates Kapha.

What to do? All the will power in the world won't stop a dried out Vata from eating vast amounts of oil to ameliorate their dryness. Usually a Kapha pacifying diet (which is dry with little oil) is recommended but such a diet aggravates Vata. The primarily approach should be to focus on pacifying vata and then the cravings for vast amounts of oily, hard to digest food will dissipate. So the approach is not to eliminate fat from the diet but instead to design a warm, moist, unctuous diet, and to gradually cut out foods and behaviors that creates dryness. (Behaviors such as drinking gallons of coffee and skipping early morning Abhyanga.)

KAPHA-PITTA CYCLE OF IMBALANCE

One of the key characteristic of Kaphas is that they are oily. They may take two showers a day and still have oily skin. When they are balanced they abhor fat. But when they become imbalanced and have accumulated too much fat and fluid and phlegm what will they need in order to get cleaned up? Heat. A body beset with fluids 'calls in' Pitta to burn off the moisture.

CYCLE OF IMBALANCE GRAPH

There is any number of cycles of imbalance. The key is to find what is at the root of the imbalance. For example, I personally, am dry and have a Vata imbalance. I need to pacify Vata. But Vata is not my primary constitution. It is the overheating (Pitta) that is the cause of the dryness. I don't disregard dealing with Vata but primarily I need to balance Pitta.

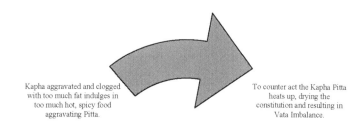

Kapha aggravated and clogged with too much fat indulges in too much hot, spicy food aggravating Pitta.

To counter act the Kapha Pitta heats up, drying the constitution and resulting in Vata Imbalance.

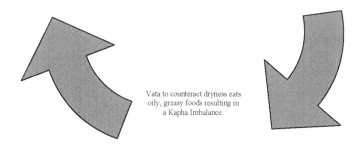

Vata to counteract dryness eats oily, greasy foods resulting in a Kapha Imbalance.

A vata physiology seeking heat might generate a Vata to Pitta cycle of imbalance. Or the coolness of Kapha could prompt a Pitta imbalance: cold seeks heat. Or a Pitta to Kapha cycle might occur: heat seeks coolness. Or a Pitta to Vata Cycle: heat and moisture seeks coolness and dryness. Or a Kapha to Vata Cycle: slowness seeks liveliness. The possible imbalances are too vast to enumerate. **The key is to understand our primary constitution and to recognize every other condition as a craving and an imbalance.** (See Graph above)

REVISITING THE QUESTIONNAIRE

If you are dubious about the accuracy of your understanding of your constitution revisit the questionnaire and consider the above information regarding imbalances. Delete questions that have been answered on the basis of an imbalance. For example question 24: Strength of digestion. Suppose you answered with a high score to item a) digestion is weak. But upon reflection you determine that this is a recent development. Most of your life you have had strong digestion. Then recognize this as an imbalance and lower your scoring for this answer.

Deleting a few answers on the basis of imbalance can change the scoring dramatically. If you were to rescore item 24 as 'strong digestion' and add that score in to the totals then the Pitta total would be considerably higher and the Vata total considerably lower. What all this means is that although you need to be concerned with weak digestion (the Vata imbalance) it is probably the result of Pitta which needs to become your primary focus. The next session focuses on how to deal with various constitutional needs and imbalances. Understanding your constitution requires careful consideration but you have the remainder of the course and ultimately as much time as you need. The remainder of this session and the next session, and particularly **Session 9: Determining Daily and Seasonal Routines** will provide further insight into understanding your Prakriti. Be patient.

CHARACTERISTICS OF THE DOSHAS REVISITED

	VATA	PITTA	KAPHA
Primary Qualities.	Movement.	Heat/Metabolism.	Structure/Fluidity.
Additional Characteristics.	Vivacity, liveliness, quick and sprightly.	Enterprising, Sharp.	Steady, stable, cautious.
Approach to life.	Quick to act.	Competitive.	Slow to take action.
Spiritual inclinations.	Joyous, blissful, ecstatic.	Compassionate, Understanding.	Devoted, devotional.
Signs of Imbalance.	Nervous, anxious, Worried.	Angry, sarcastic, Fanatical.	Depressed, lethargic, Greedy.
Tendencies when imbalanced.	Scattered. Busy, but getting little accomplished.	Domineering, Authoritarian.	Obstructive, stubborn, Childish, maudlin.
Focus in life.	Creators.	Preservers.	Stabilizers or destroyers.
Focus when imbalanced.	Let's change everything.	Let's keep the status quo no matter what.	Let's play Idi Amin.

We understand that there are over 6 billion unique constitutions on earth and the above table generalizes to provide an initial understanding of the 3 Doshas. Note that bi-doshic constitutions are more usually the case, and individuals with just one predominant dosha are not as usual. And finally, every individual is far more complex than just being a match to a simple set of general characteristics.

FURTHER UNDERSTANDING OF BODY TYPES.

To understand Kapha look to the portraits of nobility. The portraits nearly always feature individuals with large blue eyes and pale clear skin (In the case of Caucasians). It is interesting that the individuals portrayed must have approved of the artist's portrayal of themselves as aloof, arrogant and disdainful. Do the faces look down on us with compassion as might Pitta? No, it is obvious that these people took care of themselves first.

Note too, our choice of actors: Helena Bonham Carter, Sandra O, Katherine Zeta-Jones, Denzel Washington, Kate Winslet and Elizabeth Taylor. Large luminous eyes, clear skin and often a diamond shaped face. Witness also the portraits of the pharaohs, or the facial features of current world leaders. For better or worse Kaphas pretty much run the world. And while it is the most difficult dosha to get out of balance it is not a pretty sight when it does.

Vatas we may likely find immersed in the rigors of ballet or sports like ping pong that requires plenty of quickness. Seldom is a true Vata engaged in the strenuous activity of football or hockey which are the field of Pitta-Kapha and Kapha-Pitta. Note Woody Allen as a potential Vata candidate.

Pittas will gravitate towards competitive sports that are played in a cool environment: skiing, swimming and possibly golf. Note that these sports are not team sports although most NFL quarterbacks would have a high degree of Pitta.

***

EXERCISE: BALANCE FOR ME IS...

Listening to our body and giving it what it wants is key to creating good health and aging reversal. Ayurveda urges us to focus on balance and to continually expand our understanding of what balance means for us as an individual.

Now is a good time to return to your notebook and add some notes about what you need to do to maintain, or if necessary return to balance. Instead of starting afresh you might expand on the earlier writing: **Good health to me is...**For example I wrote: Balance for me is being steady and serene (more Kapha), yet being lively and vivacious (more Vata). I need to say cool and not become frazzled from overwork. I need fun and merriment and recreation. I need to eat cooling foods and surround myself with a relaxed routine and relaxed people. (Written by an individual with what type of constitution?). [18]

***

FURTHER UNDERSTANDING OF CONSTITUTION: 'DOSHAS SELDOM MARRY THEMSELVES.'

Pitta constitution seldom marries another Pitta constitution. Vata seldom marries Vata—Kapha seldom marries Kapha.

Although there are serene Pitta constitutions such as the compassionate Buddha the Dali Lama, Donald Trump is a good example of a high Pitta constitution. Often Pittas are irascible, domineering, competitive and enterprising, drivers of themselves and others.

Do Pittas marry other Pittas? Probably never. Who do they marry? Typically they marry Vata-Kaphas or Kapha-Vatas. Consider the women Mr. Trump marries: Kapha-Vatas—each looking much as if they have come out of the same mold.

Regarding couples think of the great couples of literature: Rhett Butler and Scarlett O'Hara. Othello and Desdemona. Consider the triangle described in the Great Gatsby. Daisy: Vata; her spouse Kapha (she describes him as her 'big ox'.); and Gatsby, Pitta. Enterprising and ruthless Gatsby amasses a fortune to woo Daisy away from her husband who provides for her 'stability' (a strong need for Vatas) on a level Jay Gatsby (Pitta) could never provide.

What is Katherine Zeta-Jones constitution? Who does she marry? Uberpitta, Michael Douglas.

We think we have a choice and we do. If we are Vata we have a wide choice of Pitta-Kaphas or Kapha-Pittas. And Pitta and Kapha are similarly attracted to individuals who will provide balance for them.

While Bill and Hillary Clinton both have drive and fire they are two quite different constitutions. If Hillary Clinton were to remarry she would remarry another high Pitta individual. It doesn't mean that Hillary doesn't have huge competitiveness and drive—she obliviously does—but her basic constitution is Kapha-Vata. Possibly she is close to being tri-doshic but she needs a high Pitta individual in her life, as Bill needs the steadying influence, and vivacity of Hillary's Kapha and Vata.

Barack Obama is likely tridoshic, his Pitta and Vata a bit more dominant than Kapha. He calls Michelle, who has plenty of Kapha, his rock.

Did Jesus know about Ayurveda? Most certainly: Upon this rock (Peter) I will build my church and the winds (Vata) and waters (Pitta) of time shall not prevail against it.

Did the Greeks at one time understand Ayurveda? Certainly. Many times the wisdom of Ayurveda has been revived. What a blessing to have it well understood once again.

Neurolingistics

Vata, Pitta and Kapha have different learning styles. They each respond better to, as well as speak, a different sensory language than individuals with differing constitutions.

Vatas are auditory learners. A good question for them is "How does that sound to you?", or they might say "I like the sound of that."

Pittas are often visual and are often into the sense of touch. "Do you see?" "I don't like the looks of that."

Kaphas can be into touch, "That rubs me the wrong way." but usually taste and smell resonate most highly for them. "Slow down, I need to digest that." "I don't like the smell of that." "That left a bad taste in my mouth."

SESSION WRAP-UP

Focus for the Week

Notice in yourself and your associates the influence of the three doshas.

Continue to focus on understanding your basic constitution, and continue to understand your imbalances.

Editorial Rant

Just as the study and understanding of human character is a lifetime endeavor so is the understanding our own unique make up.

It is easy to mistake an imbalance for primary constitution and this mistake should be explained by Ayurvedic practitioners to their clients though it seldom is. Pitta with a Vata imbalance will often conclude that they are Vata; Kapha often think they are Pitta; Vata often think they are tiny Kaphas.

In addition Pitta, the type A dosha, is often considered as the 'dosha of choice'. (Usually by pittas) What a pittaesque concept! Each dosha has their strengths and challenges "I yam what I yam." says Popeye. And to paraphrase Hamlet: "What a piece of work is man…" How fortunate it is that we have the variety of outlooks and abilities each of us contributes to the mix.

AGING REVERSAL

- Every aspect of our lives is important to our balance and well being.
- Our need for balance plays a key role in our choices: our spouse, where we live, what we eat, where we work, our recreation and so forth.

FURTHER READING

Though the concept of Vikriti is understood by writers on the subject of Ayurveda most often imbalance is treated as though it were the main problem. A Vata imbalance that results from Pitta Constitution being imbalanced needs to be treated but also Pitta, the root of the problem, needs the primary attention otherwise the individual will be dealing with Vata indefinitely. I don't know of any book that explains this approach to creating balance as well as it is explained here. Ain't I smart! And aren't you lucky!

FURTHER WRITING

Are you currently trapped in a cycle of imbalance? Write how you think you should deal with the imbalance and share it with your group.

Or compare some aspect of your physiology—sleeping, diet, etc.—with how it was 20 years ago. What could be done to regain excellent sleep? Remembering and writing about a great night sleep may help.

***

Session 8: *Spicing up Your Life* has some tasty recipes and suggestions for nutritional Life supporting cooking. The session will assist in further clarifying your understanding of your constitution.

Session 8
Cooking Basics: Spicing Up Your Life.

AN AYURVEDIC PROVERB:

Without proper diet, medicines are of no use;
With proper diet, medicines are of no need.

Food is medicine. Taste is the most effective of the senses for bringing balance to the doshas.

TEA

Earlier in the course a tea recipe was recommended for first thing in the morning. This tea is suitable for any time of day—particularly for Vata Constitution or those with a Vata imbalance.

- Place a slice(s) of ginger root, a piece of a cinnamon stick, cardamom pods or seeds in previously boiled water and bring to a boil. (If you prefer making the tea by using ground spices then use them.)
- Add licorice root or licorice root powder.
- If preferred, flavor the tea with lemon or lime to suit your taste.
- Brew the tea to suit your taste.

Kapha constitution may prefer more ginger and decide to use powdered ginger. Pepper as an early morning taste may make most people cringe but an individual with a predominately Kapha Constitution may lap it up. Kapha may want to increase the cardamom content, lower or omit some of the other spices and may find lime preferable to lemon.

Pitta constitution may prefer more cinnamon and/ or licorice root and may want to add nutmeg and/or fenugreek. The ginger content may be lowered for Pitta. Fenugreek seeds soaked in water make a satisfying drink for Pitta. The water used to soak the seeds may be mixed with the tea. Pittas may also eat the soaked fenugreek seeds if so inclined.

Vata constitution may prefer more licorice root and/or cinnamon, and/or an addition of fenugreek though it has a bitter taste. Salt may be an interesting addition for some Vatas. Vata may find lemon juice preferable to lime. [19]

Pre-blended teas are available but making your own allows you to create a taste which better suits your needs and taste requirements which often change with the seasons.

'APPLE PIE' FOR BREAKFAST

This recipe may be found in the book *The Answer to Cancer* by Sharma, et.al. It is a commonly recommended Ayurvedic start to the day.

- Peel and core and slice 1 organic apple (or pear) per person (sweet or sour to suit). In addition to a tasty, nutritious start to the day the effect of the meal is to provide an early morning 'bath and shower' for the alimentary canal. Although the peels have nutrients the key to value of this dish is for it to be easy to digest. If you enjoy the peels then eat the peels. If you know intellectually that you should eat the peels then who is running the show? [20] Go with what your body has to say on the matter.

- Use, plus or minus, one cup of water per fruit to suit your taste. (Less water makes a sweeter juice. All water for cooking should be pre-boiled to help remove chlorine etc.)

- Add three whole cloves per fruit. Would 4 or 5 cloves be permitted? Yes. Would 2 be okay? Yes! Would 6 be okay? Let your taste buds decide. (The cloves may be put in a tea caddy for easy retrieval, or may be inserted into the fruit where they will be less likely to be accidentally eaten. Do you like to eat them? So do I. As a boy I used to pluck them out of the baked ham and eat them greedily. [21])

- Would you like to add raisins? Figs? Dates? Prunes? Cinnamon, nutmeg, fenugreek? It's allowed.

- Soak the dried fruit and cloves etc. in the water over night if you prefer. (The apple or pear also may be left overnight covered in water if you are going to be short of time in the morning. See **Session 11: Life**. Don't rush, particularly in the morning as it sets the tone for the entire day. Practice the Go Slow Game: See **Session 14: Games**).

- Bring this fabulous breakfast treat to boiling and then turn off the heat and let it sit until the apple is 'fork tender', or cooked to suit your taste.

- If you must have coffee and toast, or bacon and eggs, or steak and flapjacks, then have them one-half hour after eating the apple.

PORRIDGE: OATS OR BARLEY?

The key to breakfast, aside from the nutritional value, is to keep the appetite satisfied until lunch. By lunchtime it is good to be pleasantly ravenous and then to begin lunch right at noon—solar noon. (See **Session 9: Daily Routines.**)

If you need a little more food than the apple dish to keep you topped up until noon try the following.

- Vata may enjoy a few peeled almonds, or oatmeal cooked with spices and dried fruit (that has been soaked in water), and cooked in milk instead of water. (No salt with milk.)
- Pitta may enjoy a date shake as dates have a cooling effect. (It is interesting how food found in the arctic is generally heating, and food from the desert is generally cooling. Can you imagine if dates had a heating effect. Would a person who lived in the desert want to eat them? It must have been quite the whirlwind that went through the proverbial junkyard to create this 747 on which we are floating around the sun.)
- Kapha may enjoy barley flakes cooked up similar to oatmeal. Barley is light. A wee bit of honey and skim milk may be suitable. Cardamom may provide a pleasing taste and counteract the 'sticky' effects of the milk. Kaphas cook the barley flakes in water, not milk. If honey fires up the

appetite then use it in lassi (See **Appendix A**) after the main meal, or in some other way.

Variety is the spice of life. Create variety in all your meals.

JIFFY DAHL

Dahl is an East Indian dish made with lentils or mung dahl.

From an Ayurvedic perspective the spices should be cooked in both oil and water as our body's cells have both oil and water permeable membranes. (Most Chinese Food is cooked in both oil and water.)

To begin: Along with ghee (especially for Pittas) or olive oil, or oil that you prefer, add your spices to a high quality stainless steel pan or pot. Sauté the spices lightly until you smell the pleasant aroma. If you wish to include mustard seeds you may want to 'pop' them by sautéing them in the ghee prior to adding the spices. To do this add ghee to the pan, cover and heat the seeds on a medium heat until they pop'. Shake the pan as if making popcorn. Ghee has high heat tolerance but it will scorch.

Take the pan off the heat in order to cool it just enough add water. Experiment with 5 parts water to 1 part dahl.

- Add the dahl. (Make sure it is clean and free of seeds or stones.)
- Add salt later, but prior to the dahl being cooked. Ditto for turmeric if you like extra turmeric.
- Combine 2 grains. [22] In this recipe I am going to use red lentils and quinoa. Both of these grains cook in about the same amount of time so add them at the same time. (Some grains may take

longer than others to cook so add one, then the faster cooking grain later.)

- Add the vegetables. Carrots and cabbage cook in about the same length of time. Carrots and broccoli would require that the carrots go in first and the broccoli later. [23] (Both partially cooked and mushy vegetables are frowned upon.)

When the dish is ready to remove from the heat add greens such as cilantro, cress, or Italian parsley. Chopped dulse, purple in color, raisins (revered in Ayurveda) and some cashews or other nuts sprinkled on top further enhance the taste, nutrition and make for an attractive presentation.

RAW FOOD

Ayurveda recommends that most individuals have some raw food every day. Some constitutions with stronger digestion may have more raw food than those with weaker digestion. Ayurveda sees one of the functions of cooking as the enlivening of the Life of the food. While Ayurveda promotes the idea that we should follow what our body wants, most Ayurvedic practitioners would ask a person who eats a large portion of their food raw if the body was relishing that food or in fact they were eating on the basis of their intellect.

JIFFY SOUP

Jiffy soup may be made in similar fashion to dahl only using more liquid. (Whey, a left over from making Paneer, may be used as the stock for soup). Once cooked the dish may be put in blender to create a thick soup. Sprinkle with a pleasing garnish.

LASSI: A DELIGHTFUL YOGURT DRINK

What to drink? **Lassi** [24] is a drink made with yogurt mixed with water. If you wish add honey (or raw sugar) and saffron. Or try it with salt and toasted cumin. Simply divine!

COOKING FOR COUPLES

As noted earlier, individuals within a couple are seldom (and probably never) the same dosha and seldom have the same taste requirements. Some couples have a dosha in common: Vata-Pitta and Kapha-Pitta have Pitta constitution in common for example. But single doshic individuals who team up with bidoshic individuals (which is often the case) may have problems.

- ***Vata teams up with a Pitta-Kapha or Kapha-Pitta:***

If the Vata cooks, they likely favor predominately sour and salty tastes as well as unctuous and heavy dishes. The Kapha-pitta spouse has trouble with this food. Sour aggravates Pitta, and oily and heavy qualities are the last thing Kapha needs. On the other hand if the Kapha-Pitta cooks, then the food tends to be dry and light and either spicy with jalapenos and curries or bland to suit pitta.

- ***A Pitta teams up with Vata-Kapha:***

If the Pitta cooks, the food is cooling. If the Vata-Kapha cooks, the food is warming or possibly atomic hot, spicy, and possibly loaded with garlic and onions.

What to do? Get a new partner? From an Ayurvedic perspective one may marry a different person but their constitution will likely be pretty much the same as that of the first spouse. The answer (to the food issue) is to create a spice mix(es) that are suitable for each individual and to heat the spices in ghee until the aroma is first noticeable and then to drizzle the mixture on one's food. Second, a variety of foods to satisfy each of the six tastes should be available at the main meal of the day.

SALT

Add salt into the food prior to the cooking being complete. Adding salt at the table after the food has been cooked is not practiced in most traditional cultures. Salt cooked in the food is thought to be more easily assimilated.

It is unbelievable that even our salt has been bleached! Avoid chlorine and additives. Unpolluted salt from ancient deposits found in deep mines may be the best choice considering the condition of our earth's environment.

MILK

Milk is revered in Ayurveda as the best of foods. The thinking is that everyone should have at least a bit of milk everyday—lacto intolerance is considered to be a sign of an imbalance. But if you can't stomach milk here are some recommendations.

Boiling milk before drinking is recommended by Ayurveda though some research purports to show that boiling destroys valuable nutrients. I boil milk prior to drinking it.

Whole milk that is not homogenized is thought to be the best milk.[25] Homogenized milk is considered to be more difficult to digest. Adding whipping cream to skim milk may be a way to get 'whole milk'.

Is the Vitamin D added to the milk synthetic? Ayurveda frowns on synthetics of any sort. Who doesn't—except the milk marketers and their mad 'scientists'?

Store milk in something other than plastic as toxins from the plastic are often fat soluble.

A cup of warm milk is recommended prior to bed. The warm milk will help bring on sleep. If one drinks the milk and waits more than a half hour to go to bed the effect of the milk will be to keep one awake. In addition to promoting sleep, warm milk provides hydration and isn't as likely to send one staggering to the loo in the middle of the night. (This is also part of the reason for the recommendation of soupy dahl or soup for supper.) Warm milk spiced with cardamom is delicious and will help counteract mucus if this is a concern. Cinnamon and ginger are also fabulous with warm milk. Any of these spices may be added in any combination and proportion.

Milk may be combined with sweet tastes but is generally not recommended with foods which have sour and salty tastes. For example, milk based chowders are not recommended.

If you have trouble drinking or ingesting milk add one cup of milk to one cup of water, add turmeric and black pepper and boil the mixture down to one cup. Strain the mixture and enjoy. This can also be a great mid- morning or mid-afternoon tonic for people who enjoy milk. How much pepper and turmeric should you use? As in any Ayurvedic recipe: season to suit your taste.

CURDS AND WHEY

Paneer (see **Appendix C**) is the curds (the basis for cheese) separated from the whey by heating the milk and adding yogurt and/or lime or lemon juice. For commercial use the whey is powdered and sold to body builders who eat it in order to build muscle. Liquid whey is also rich in protein and tasty, and may be used as a stock for soup or dahl. It is considered by Ayurveda to be hard to digest as well as heavy and clogging. Use it only if your digestion is strong, and monitor how you feel after eating a meal made with this product. I love the stuff.

LEFTOVERS

Session 11: Life makes the point that food has Life in it. Heating food enlivens the Life but once the food cools the Life dissipates. Leftovers are not recommended. What to do?

If you must eat leftovers reheat them with ghee and also include some fresh food in the meal. Fresh fruit and vegetables provide the best source of Life. Reheating these is less acceptable than reheating grains. Grains are often stored for years and have a great ability to hold on to Life and are probably more acceptable reheated. Milk products such as paneer, yogurt and the like may be stored in the fridge, though fresh every day is thought to be best. Ghee may be stored unrefrigerated for a very long time (assuming bits of toast crumbs and the like don't end up in it.) Raisins are praised in Ayurveda as an excellent food yet they are 'old' and have been 'heated' when they were dried. Go figure how this works, but nonetheless we know intuitively that fresh is best.

In addition to the Life in leftover food being depleted the food may become a 'poison'. Notice particularly garnishes such as parsley that have been sprinkled on top of a dish a few minutes before serving. These seem to be extremely unpalatable when served at the next meal.

For us to be filled with Life, and to avoid being filled with something other than Life, it may be good practice to skip the leftovers.

A SUGGESTED ORDERING OF THE TASTES.

In various Ayurvedic tomes one may find a proposed ordering of tastes to be followed as one eats a meal. (See **Session 2**) Sweet is considered to be the first taste to eat. This makes sense as sweets—meat, bread, butter, etc—are heavy and the most difficult to digest. In addition, eating them right away gets the blood sugar requirements balanced and being satisfied in this regard may result in all the sooner being less hungry and eating less. A small sweet at the beginning of the meal—for example a small piece of carrot cake, no frosting—might be just enough sugar to result in a more leisurely and satisfying meal. Sometimes I eat red grapes and cashews. Honey and cream is also a yummy way to start.

HOW WE EAT, IS AS IMPORTANT AS WHAT WE EAT.

If you were to think back on your eating experiences—both the good ones and the not so good ones—you could come up with (and probably have) a common sense list of dos and don'ts at meal time. Consider:

- Are we comfortable in a noisy restaurant, served by a rushed, abrasive waiter?
- Our best meals have probably been leisurely, and taken in relaxing, clean and pleasant surroundings.
- Ever had a great meal when you were angry or worried?
- If there is an emotional disruption just prior to a meal wait for the physiology to settle before eating. Sip some water and take a short walk. Practice Darth Vader breathing.
- Have you ever had a great meal while you were still half full from the previous meal?
- Have you ever had a great meal when you were rushed? Eat slowly.

None of the above is rocket science. We know what to do; our body has been telling us how to best live since we were born. When we contravene these above approaches to eating how do we feel? The body is simply sending us a message: don't treat yourself poorly/ or treat yourself well!

In every culture there is a tradition of being thankful before and after meals. Being thankful at its best is felt in the heart. If we need to invoke a prayer, ceremony or discussion to stimulate thankfulness so be it, though the sight and smell of the food alone may invoke a flood of gratitude.

AFTER THE MEAL

After a meal you may find it agreeable to lie on your left side and rest. Rest is a great assist to digestion given that the body is devoting a large portion of its energy and blood supply to heating and digesting the food (particularly if one has washed the meal down with a 32oz. blizzard gulp.) Lying on the left side allows the stomach juices to flow to the latter portions of the meal creating a chance for better digestion.

If you have an acid reflux problem then lying back at a 45 degree angle may mitigate the upflow of acidic materials, as will following the dictum that one should eat only until about three-quarters full. These recommendations may mitigate the symptoms but you need to fix whatever is causing the problem. Note the pancreas story in *Session 2.*

SESSION WRAP-UP

FOCUS FOR THE WEEK

- If you don't drink milk try to find a way to have a bit before bed—even if it is a teaspoon in a cup of hot water. But if you can't stand the taste of milk don't drink it.
- Stay hydrated throughout the night.
- Work on incorporating spices which you find pleasant into your diet.

EDITORIAL RANT

The portrayal of meals as somehow similar to fueling a car rampant on TV—particularly on 'cop shows'—is just more of the destructive nonsense our culture is teaching our children and spreading throughout the planet. Food is a gift for the well being of the systems within us and ultimately for our self. The aroma of food as well as the texture and visual appeal **prepare** the physiology to digest and assimilate the nutrition and the Life of the food. Though I hope for an age of enlightenment if the understanding of Life portrayed on TV keeps deteriorating I'm sure we will have kids with zippers installed on their stomachs so mom can unzip them and slip in a pouch of goop in order to give them a 'good warm start to the day'.

Aging Reversal
- Maintaining ample hydration throughout the night is important.
- How we eat is as important as what we eat.
- Nutritious, satisfying cooking can be fun and simple.

Further Reading

I have a library of cookbooks but not one of them that I like enough to recommend strongly. See **Reading:** Banchek as possibly the best.

It is not just the six tastes that require balance but the textures and stimulation of all the senses. Ayurveda understands that foods should be cooked and served with compatible foods. If you have a cookbook that bases its recipes on this ancient understanding of food I would like to hear about it. What I have done is to rely on my body's intelligence to direct me as to what to cook. This approach can work quite well.

Further Writing

Best meal ever.
Most fun cooking experience.

***

Session 9: Daily and Seasonal Routines is an opportunity to get into sync with the Nature.

Session 9
Daily, Seasonal And Lifetime Cycles

MAKE CHANGES GRADUALLY

Abrupt change can create a shock that the body will eventually need to repair. The 'cold turkey' approach to quitting smoking—or sugar, caffine, or anything else—is an opportunity to create an experience from hell. Do we need more stress in our lives? Ayurveda recommends gradual change.

What to do? What to do?

LEAVING BAD HABITS BEHIND

- First, find out what the body 'gets' from the habit. Is it fat's energy or a specific taste as examples?
- Meet the need in a Life supporting way.
- Let the poor behavior gradually 'fall off'.

Be easy with yourself. I doubt any one of us, one day tucked under the sheets in the 'Shady Glen Old Folks' Home' is going to be complaining that we didn't have enough stress in our life. *Session 15: Trauma* includes a technique for dealing with cravings, and we will discuss further in *Session 10: Vedic Exercise*, how to avoid the 'No pain no gain', and 'Cold Turkey' practices which are destructive to physiology.

THE DAILY CYCLE OF HUMAN PHYSIOLOGY

At dawn the world awakens. We also should be awake—and out of bed.

From dawn forward, the daylight part of the day is divided into 3 sections the first having the qualities of Kapha, the second the qualities of Pitta, and the third the qualities of Vata. It is convenient to designate these as being from 6am to 10 am, 10am to 2pm, and 2pm to 6 pm but these times are seldom accurate at the higher latitudes or during daylight savings time. Given that many of us live a distance from the center of the time zones (where it is solar noon at noon) our 'man made' time is out of sync with solar time. You must adjust time on the basis of the time of year, your location in your time zone, and possibly daylight savings time. This is not a great challenge, nor does the accuracy need to be scrupulously precise. Noon is when the sun is at its zenith. Divide the time from sunrise to sunset by 3 to find the length of each of the three time period and then determine the Vata, Pitta, Kapha times of day. (The length of the day and subsequently the length of the time periods will vary the higher your location in the northern or southern latitudes and depending upon the time of year.)

Do we have an urge to spring out of bed at 6 in the morning during the dark of winter? Probably not. In summer does one have an urge to crawl into bed at 10 o'clock at night when the sun is shining? Probably not. The time periods, depending on the time of year, will expand or contract in length.

The First Kapha Time of Day begins at dawn and continues for one third of the daylight hours. Pitta Time of Day then begins: half of it prior to solar noon and half after. Then Vata Time begins and is complete at sunset.

The second Kapha time of day is the first 1/3rd of the time from sunset to dawn. Pitta governs the second 1/3rd and Vata the 1/3rd ending at dawn. If you have been listening to your body throughout your life you are aware that the 'quality of time' changes during these different times of day.

The key to performing the most effective action in each of these time periods is held in the phrase, *the characteristics of the Doshas are lively during the time of day they govern.* For example the pre-dawn world is alive with movement. This Vata time of day (night really) has a lively, energetic quality to it.

ACTIVITY RECOMMENDED FOR THE SIX DAILY TIME PERIODS

The activities recommended on the basis of the six daily time periods may be adjusted to suit individual constitutions. A Vata constitution may wish to rest at the end of the day (Vata time of day) whereas Kapha or Pitta may find this a suitable time for work or exercise, or creative work.

Predawn Vata is the proper time of day to arise. Waking up and getting out of bed prior to dawn during the Vata Time of Day sets a lively tone within the physiology for the entire day. One carries the quality of the time of day at which they arise: Vata—lively; Kapha—sluggish; and Pitta grumpy.

The Vata Time of day is a time for washing and cleaning the body. A complete evacuation the bowel is recommended. See **Session 17: The Mud and the Lotus.** Vata time is a good time for Yoga Postures, Prayer and Meditation.

A light breakfast including fruit (moist, sweet and heavy which pacify Vata) is recommended in the morning.

FROM THE POET RUMI

> The breeze at dawn has secrets to tell you
> Don't go back to sleep.
> You must ask for what you really want
> Don't go back to sleep.

We snooze we lose. Early to bed early to rise, etc… these sayings make sense from an Ayurvedic perspective.

THE QUALITY OF THE CUSPS

It is important to note that the time immediately preceding and following a time period 'colours' or flavors the last hour and first hour of those time periods. For example the first hour of the Kapha Time has a Vata quality to it; the last hour of Kapha Time has a Pitta quality; the first hour of the Pitta has a Kapha quality and so forth.

The first Kapha Time of Day, in the morning from dawn until about 10 a.m, is the best time of day for exercise and work as Kapha promotes strength and endurance.

Kapha's influence will carry into the First Pitta Time of day which begins around 10 am and work may continue until noon, but one should eat the large meal of the day at noon or shortly after. Rest briefly or as needed (but don't sleep) after the meal, plan the remainder of the day and return to work. Pitta constitution, susceptible to heat may not feel like working until well into the Vata time of day and at that time may find a second wind.

THE SECOND HALF OF THE DAY

The afternoon, the shank end of the day, is dominated by Vata. A person with predominantly Vata Constitution may not feel strong during this time. Light activity, study and meditation are recommended although stronger constitutions may find work and vigorous activity enjoyable.

The second Kapha time of day from sunset to about 10 pm is a time for merriment. A pleasant walk after a light, savory super is good for all constitutions. [26] Family time and pleasant life supporting entertainment are recommended. Kapha's jovial nature is predominant during this time of day. Enjoy!

Pitta time begins around 10 pm. It is signified by the proverbial 'second wind'. Don't let the second wind whisk you into activity. Be in bed before the second Pitta Time of Day begins. If you are in bed sleeping during this time the immune system will have the energy to clean the physiology of impurities. If you become immersed in work instead of sleeping the immune system will miss this opportunity to clean and heal the physiology. If you can't sleep then just lay there passively giving the immune system the chance to do what it does so well.

In addition don't overload the body with a large meal or stimulating activity prior to this time period. Let the body sleep and repair itself and get ready for the coming day. This recommendation is possibly more important than either getting up before dawn, or eating the main meal at noon. It is absolutely crucial for good health to allow the body to clean and repair itself. But having established an early bedtime into one's routine does not preclude the occasional late meal or night of celebration. In most traditional cultures the full moon is a time for celebration and festival.

THE DAY BEGINS THE NIGHT BEFORE

There is a dictum in Ayurveda that states that 'the day begins the night before'. Your sleep and the repair it provides are needed for the coming day. The noon meal of the previous day fuels your body during the coming day. The bowel movement before dawn is to a large degree contingent upon having eaten a light savory supper, remaining properly hydrated throughout the night and getting to sleep prior to the second Pitta Time of day.

To try to create a 'good day' beginning the morning of that day is at best minimally effective. At worst we see people relying on stimulants and pain killers to 'pull them through the day'. How sad.

SEASONAL CYCLES

The Fall season in many parts of the world is usually a windy, dry time of year. Cold, dry weather aggravates Vata.

The cold and damp of the Winter and the Spring seasons aggravate Kapha Dosha.

Summer heat and humidity aggravate Pitta Dosha.

These seasonal effects vary greatly around the world. For example winter on the prairies is dry and windy—aggravating Vata Dosha more so than Kapha. In other parts of the world—the arctic or Indonesia for example the Spring and Fall seasons may scarcely noticeable. When I was traveling in Africa during their 'winter' people were wearing toques and sweaters in the 'cool' 75 degree (22C) weather. Our body cries out for us to make adjustments to our diet and lifestyle in order to ameliorate the effects of the seasons. The key to these seasonal concepts is to know what weather aggravates (and pacifies) which dosha and to adjust our lifestyle to the weather. We each know the weather that aggravates our unique constitution. It is more likely that listening to the preferences of our physiology will provide more reliable info than that determined from the results of our questionnaire. Continue to pay close attention to messages from your physiology as you work through *The Aging Reversal Course.* Determine what your unique constitution requires during the various weather of the year.

In Fall (dry, windy conditions) moist, unctuous foods; oil massage; saunas, steam baths and a calm environment away from the wind help pacify Vata.

In Winter and Spring, (cool, moist conditions) lighter, dryer foods; brightness, sunshine, light and stimulation will be appreciated as each of these help pacify Kapha.

In Summer (hot, humid conditions) cooling foods; swimming, walking at night when the air is cool are the order of the season to pacify Pitta.

DIFFERENT SEASONS MAY BE PLEASIN'

One season may be heaven for one constitution, and for another hell. A Vata or Kapha person with a shortage of Pitta may love summer; or a Pitta person with a shortage of Kapha may come alive in winter. The needs of our unique physiology and the effects of the seasonal variations require our attention. In this regard we need to design proper routine and lifestyle. [27]

SEASONAL CLEANSING

During each season an excess of the dosha aggravated by the weather of that season may accumulate within the body. By the time of the change to the next season the body may be dealing with this imbalanced dosha plus facing the challenge of adjusting to the new weather conditions. For example, after the heat of Summer there may be a need to balance Pitta as well to prepare for the cool dry weather of Fall. The often heard comment that someone is sick because of a change in the seasons or a change of the weather makes sense from an Ayurvedic perspective.

Ayurveda recommends Pancha Karma three times a year at the change of each season. PK treatments are for the most part divine: warm herbalized oil massage; steam treatment; nasal inhalations; deep tissue massage; herbalized paste massages; herbalized steam baths; eye treatments; and internal cleansing are a few of the wide variety of modalities employed. While it is easy to get focused on the pleasantness of the experience it is also interesting to remember that these treatments are supporting health and the reversing aging by cleaning the body of impurities. In a proactive and exceedingly pleasant (there's that word again) way Panchakarma follows the same lead as that of our body as it reacts to sickness. When sick we stay warm; eat less; rest; sweat and throw off toxins—exactly what Panchakarma does in a proactive and enjoyable way.[28] What a great way to deal with the buildup of imbalance and to promote wellness. [29]

The length of PK session may vary in the West from as little as 3 days to months with the usual session lasting one week. The lifestyle during this time is best summed up as one of luxury and rest accompanied by warm, savory, unctuous food, and plenty of interesting and uplifting but restful activity.

PK is a time to deal with the impurities accumulated during the previous season. These toxins need to be eliminated or we face the danger of them building up season after season, collecting deep within the tissues and interfering with the body's memory of how to accurately rebuild itself.

It would indeed require an exceptional physiology to remain toxin free while not having had access to PK. Our world is awash in synthetic toxins that no living organism is immune to. By a very young age our physiology begins to be unable to deal with this inundation, and toxicity begins to build up particularly in the fat tissues and organs. PK, through heating, oiling and massaging, is extremely effective at removing toxins from the physiology.

PK PREP

The time prior to PK is the time to prepare the body for the session. Light unctuous food is recommended along with living as stress free a life as possible. During this time—usually four or more days—progressively increasing amounts of ghee are consumed. Ghee loosens up the toxins, particularly those within the digestive track, and as important, protects the lining of the digestive track from particularly corrosive toxins that may be released during the PK treatments. On the night before PK begins a mild laxative is taken. While this flushes out the toxins that have been loosened the ghee continues to coat and protect the digestive track.

In addition, to the week of PK Prep and the week of PK treatments, there will be encouragement to live a particularly Satvic lifestyle for at least a few weeks after the PK session. For maximum benefit one should commit to at least a month of ultra healthy living both prior to and after the treatments.

In Lieu of PK

Certainly what could be easily done at the change of seasons is to set aside a week and during that time stay warm, rested, and eat light unctuous food. In addition before beginning the week one could try the ghee prep and laxative. To follow this routine would take about the same amount of time needed to recover from a cold or flu—and is a lot more pleasant. [30]

Although there are cleanses available on the market I haven't seen one that I would recommend. It is certain that most cleanses have the ability to loosen up impurities but do they have the ability to remove the impurities from the body? And more important do they provide a means of protection for the inner physiology during the cleanse? I've seen no recognition of this problem from the manufacturers of cleanses. The intense heat of some cleanses may inflict serious damage to the physiology. A cleanse without protection for the digestive system is not recommended.

LIFETIME CYCLES

Youth is a time when Kapha dominates. Youths are usually strong, flexible, and energetic with great stamina and endurance. But youth may be subject to sniffles (kapha imbalance), and during times of growth may be lethargic, and depressed during the teenage years (kapha imbalance).

Adulthood to middle-age is dominated by Pitta. Adults often have 'fire in the belly' and may be enterprising and aggressive and are usually immersed in careers.

After middle age Vata is more predominant. We may be more blissful and joyful. We may gravitate towards creative pursuits. Vata imbalances such as dry skin, interrupted sleep and a lack of strength and endurance may be features of these years.

A person of Kapha Constitution may do well in the Vata time of life (the elder years) as may Pitta, whereas Vata who may have enjoyed strength and fluidity of kapha during early life, may find the difficulties of Vata exacerbated during the Vata years.

Any scenario is possible. During childhood one may have been sickly, and later in life become a picture of health. Or one may have been weak during their middle years and find that their elder years are the best part of life. The possibilities are too vast to enumerate.

Over the millennia few people would have had any instructional manual other than information from their physiology. Today we shouldn't be timid about using information from our physiology. It shouldn't be a concern if what your body wants is not considered 'normal': breathing cold air from the freezer, or sipping hot water while the outside temperature is 100 degrees F. What works for you is 'normal'. Whatever your body needs is what it needs. The only corollary to this dictum is that we meet these needs in a 'Life supporting' manner.

SESSION WRAP-UP

FOCUS FOR THE WEEK

- Focus on and redesign daily routine to meets the needs of your constitution throughout the changing circumstances of life.

- Throughout **The Aging Reversal Course** each of us has been writing an instruction manual of what works for them. You have gathered information from two sources: the information your body provides and the course information. Now, at the end of this session, is a good time to put forth more effort and continue to develop your personal instructional manual for your constitution in your **I R Healthy** notebook.

EDITORIAL RANT

What our children see on TV advertizing is often complete nonsense. A 'hot' looking chick fires back a painkiller and says in a sexy voice "You don't know the power of 'el dopa'." She then joyously dives into a pool and has a rigorous early morning swim after which she sails through her day. What kind of an approach to life and well being is this? What are we teaching our children?

By way of contrast it is easy to sail through the day when we meet the needs of human physiology and treat the body well. With the body satisfied and well prepared we can enjoy the swim without painkillers—a message we are unlikely to see on TV.

AGING REVERSAL

- Our body has different demands throughout the daily, seasonal, and lifetime cycles. We need to develop a lifestyle best suited to our unique physiology in order to meet the needs created by the conditions of these varying times.
- Our body is intuitively aware of the cycles of nature. When we heed these 'Laws of Nature' Nature supports us. When we disregard these

cycles the body requires an expenditure of energy.

Most books on Ayurveda have sections on designing routine though they are not as clear about the variations, cusps and overlap of the time cycles as found in this course. Lucky you.

FURTHER WRITING

Describe a time of day when you were deeply aware of the quality of time. The energy of the early morning before dawn. The need to get into bed and sleep before 10 pm. Strong appetite at noon. The stillness between the time periods or seasons.

***

Next is **Session 10: Vedic Exercise**. There is much in this coming session that our body already intuitively understands. Imagine an exercise program designed to produce euphoria!

Session 10
Vedic Exercise

RE—CREATION

As children we played and laughed and played some more. Proper exercise rejuvenates and fills our physiology with exuberance and joy and helps re create physiology. The usual pronunciation of the word—*wreck re ation*—is a quite apt description of most exercise programs. But consider the prefix and the root of the word recreation—re and create. Exercise recreates. Improper exercise creates toxins and drives them into the tissues: proper exercise loosen and remove existing debris from the body.

Vasant Lad's book *The Science of Self-Healing* listed in the **Reading and Websites** proposes the idea that Ayurveda was originally created for Yogi's because of their need to release the toxins loosened up through their Yogic practices. This may have been the case but in my view any human being, given that physiology always seeks balance, is capable of releasing toxicity. While release of toxins is a requirement for Karma Yogis[31] major stress release can occur in any individual. This phenomenon is not specific to Yogi's particularly given the current pollution level of the planet. Ayurveda and Vedic Exercise are essential to good health and aging reversal in that they assist in cleaning and purifying the body. (See **Session 14: The Millstones**)

GUIDELINES

Maintaining the following guidelines during exercise is essential to avoid straining the body and exercise is most effective when these instructions are followed.

- 'Do less and accomplish more.' Train at 50% of your maximum. 70% of max and higher will not work in the long term as it creates damage and aging.
- If your body is stressed—that is to say you feel unwell—skip the exercise session for that day.
- Build up an oxygen surplus prior to exercise.
- Maintain the surplus during exercise.
- Get into the 'zone' as you warm up.

There is no sense trying to practice Vedic Exercise if you are going to skimp on these instructions. Stressing the body will produce the same sad results as the 'no pain no gain' and 'feel the burn' schools of exercise. Why bother?

PREPARATION FOR EXERCISE

Effective breathing, proper hydration, proper eating habits, diet, abhyanga, listening to the body, all described earlier in Sessions 1 to 9 is an excellent basis upon which to build a Life supporting exercise program

***

Notebook Exercise

Return to your **I R Healthy** notebook and list the number of exercise programs you have tried over the course of your life. Consider such topics as: How long were you able to endure each attempt? Why did you stop? What percentage of your life have you been involved in an exercise program? How did the program make you feel in terms of energy and vitality?

Don't be concerned about the failure of these programs but instead figure out what your body didn't approve of, and delete these features from your new program. Also particularly note the types of exercise you enjoyed and were able to maintain.

Also add to your notebook a time when you felt light and invigorated during and after exercise. And sketch out what you want to feel during and after your new program. Describe the level of fitness you wish to have. This is really an extension of the original question of 'Health to me is…?' Writing gives you time think about what you want, and allows the idea to be introduced into and supported by consciousness.

***

STRAIN AND PAIN EQUALS NO GAIN

Exercise, as commonly practiced strains the body. From professional and Olympic athletes, to our youth in minor hockey, 'no pain no gain' exercise drives toxins deep within the tissues and is destructive to physiology. The pseudoscience of a vitamin supplement, or the 'power' of a pain reliever isn't going to change the fact that the body needs to recover from the abuse it has suffered over the years. Eventually a strained body will find a way to stop the abuse. And whether deterioration is blamed on poor genetics, or on a lack of guts, the body inevitably revolts, requiring us to stop the pain, and take the time to rest and heal. In the extreme this slowing down is euphemistically called 'old age'.

PROPER EXERCISE ROUTINE

Ideally, you are up and out of bed before dawn and by following the instructions in **Session 2**, you are well hydrated, hygiene has been taken care of, abhyanga has been enjoyed, you have done breathing exercises in the fresh predawn air, performed yoga postures or tai chi postures, performed Pranayama, (**Appendix P**) meditated, transcended into silence (**Sessions 15 and 16**) said your prayers, are neither hungry nor uncomfortably full, and you feel good. You have immensely enjoyed this warm up time as you have spent most of it 'in the moment' which is what proper exercise is designed to do—to get us into the moment. You are not rushing the various aspects of the program in order to get on with something 'fun': the entire program is fun!

By exercising when your physiology is strained you will add strain to an already challenged physiology which will require additional energy to repair. If you do not feel well then do not exercise. Rest.[32] To contravene this key principle of Vedic Exercise is a chance to create a strain deficit that will need to be repaired.

Now, after all of the above preparation, all of which you have enjoyed, you are ready to enjoy exercise.

SURYA NAMASKARA (SUN SALUTE), AND YOGA POSTURES

I don't feel comfortable 'teaching' the delicate set of Sun Salute postures through print but they are found in numerous books on Ayurveda, some of them listed in **Read-**

ing and Websites, as well as on <u>youtube</u>. The best way to learn the Sun Salute is from a competent instructor.

SELECTING A COMPETENT INSTRUCTOR

Make sure your instructor is of the 'effortless and easy' school of thought, and a person who understands that attention enlivens.

Ask questions. If the instructor is all about 'no pain, no gain' and doesn't know which postures strengthen which organs, or doesn't even know that the asanas strengthen organs, or is into power yoga, and then I encourage you to look elsewhere for an instructor.

YOGA POSTURES

Also I recommend that you find a competent instructor to design and teach you a set of Yoga Postures that are suited specifically to your needs. While I do not include a set of yoga postures in the course I do supply some valuable notions regarding the practice and benefits of yoga asanas (pronounced short a: *a za on a s*) for your consideration.

One of the well known benefits of yoga postures is that they stretch and exercise the muscles and tendons and so forth, but this is not their primary purpose.[33] The true beauty of a properly performed set of postures is that the practice of them places the internal organs in unordinary positions which results in unusual (but gentle) 'stresses' on these organs. The result is that the organs acted upon are **cleaned, strengthened** and **rested.** By practicing these postures you support your body's natural propensity to clean, strengthen and repair itself. Strengthened! Cleansing, resting and strengthening the liver, kidneys and spleen!

What a novel and seemingly odd idea! Did your phy ed coach teach you that you need to strengthen your internal organs? What folly it is to attempt to build muscles while having weak interior organs. How strong are the muscles, how long will they last and what strains accumulate in the ill prepared organs as one 'works out'?

SUN SALUTE INSTRUCTIONS (SEE ALSO APPENDIX E)

Amazingly, Surya Namaskara has become immensely popular in the West in a very short time. I wish that all the useful knowledge of the East would be as readily accepted. (For example the Child's Pose asana is of great use as an antidote to depression.)

- Face East. [34]
- The best time of day to practice the Sun Salute is in the morning but any time of day will be beneficial though the postures are not recommended to be practiced in the evening.
- Begin and end each set with the Namaste posture. (You are greeting the Sun. From a physiological point of view the Namaste is an opportunity to pause, breathe normally and rest.)
- Perform the movements smoothly much like a Tai Chi movement. No quickness or jerking. (See The Go Slow Exercise in **Session 14**.)
- No forcing.
- No straining.
- Breathing should be easy—a protocol for all Vedic Exercise.
- Mild Darth Vader breathing is quite acceptable.
- Focus on the breathing.
- Focus on the body.

- 5 seconds between postures.
- Very little time is given to the central posture— the posture where 8 points of the body touch the 'earth'. Note that the lungs have been emptied of air prior to this posture and remains so until one begins the next posture.
- Even only one set of The Sun Salute is beneficial.
- Work up gradually to several sets if this suits you—max 12.
- Keep in mind the principles of Vedic Exercise.
- Rest in the repose posture after you finish this part of the work out.
- A body scan might be a good thing to do at this point but allow the mind to attend as it will.

Though I include a set of sketches for beginners of each position in **Appendix E** find a competent instructor to teach the Sun Salute.

The benefits of this 'exercise' are probably not fully understood by anyone. Certainly the act of breathing in sync with the postures promotes mind body coordination. All major muscles are put to use. The exercise no doubt has salubrious effects on the marmas (See **Session 11: Life**) and has positive effects on the psycho, immuno, neuro, endoctrinal systems. (Referred to as PINE, See **Reading and Websites:** Gabor Mate) Check your pulse before and after your performance to see if your pulse rate has in fact decreased. Do less and accomplish more isn't just a slogan.

Now that you have completed your pre exercise routine including the brief rest after the Sun Salute you are well prepared for an enjoyable exercise session. I will now outline how to achieve peak performance without straining the physiology.

LEVEL 1: SUPER OXYGENATE THE BODY—GRADUALLY

Perhaps while walking, or easily playing whatever sport you have chosen—ping pong for example—gradually guide your body into the 'zone'. 'Workout' initially at a low level that does not cause your heart rate to exceed approximately 30 beats per minute above your resting rate. (Resting rate is your heart rate first thing in the morning.) It is difficult to believe that 30 beats per minutes above resting will be correct for everyone. For some individuals 20 bpm above resting and for others 40 bpm above resting may be what is required—experiment. Initially go with 30 bpm above your resting rate. Your body will tell you if you need to make an adjustment. Listen and trust. The key is that you are comfortable and not straining during this time of super-oxygenating your physiology.

During this initial period of exercise breathe deeply but easily with intent to build up an oxygen surplus. Once you have effortlessly done so then the trick is to easily maintain this surplus throughout your exercise session.

DETERMINING YOUR TRAINING HEART RATE

Subtract your age and add your resting heart rate to the figure 220. Divide this total in half. For you, this figure (give or take a bit depending on the advice from your physiology) is the best heart rate at which to exercise.

For example at 50% of maximum, a 60 year old with a resting heart rate of 60 would have a training rate of 110. (220 minus 60, plus 60, divided by 2)

Many athletes train at 70%, 80%, and 90% and for brief periods even at 100% of their maximum. These levels strain the physiology and cannot be maintained throughout the years even by exceptional physiologies without incurring some damage. To train at 60% may be sustainable but training at 50% will produce the same level of fitness though more time (days and months) is usually required to reach the levels reached by training at a higher heart rate.

LEVEL 2

When you feel comfortable and well oxygenated continue your workout at a level somewhere between the *Resting plus 30,* and the 50% level calculated above. (For me this is somewhere between 84 (resting pulse 54+30) and 110). During this time focus on your physiology: your breathing, heart, muscles and coordination.

LEVEL 3

After a time (which might be as much as 15 minutes or more, but it could occur right away) and everything seems smooth and effortless and you notice that you are in the zone then gradually increase your activity up to the level of your ideal training rate. Don't crank up the level of activity hoping to get into the zone: instead get into the zone and gently move to your ideal training rate. Once there, if you find that your breathing becomes labored, or a muscle begins to ache or other discomforts occur then slow the pace and focus on that area of concern until things smooth out. (Attention heals.)

I understand that to not push is counter to everything I was brought up to believe. My urge is to 'push through the pain'. My thought is that 'my dumb body is holding me back from having fun'. Please remember that in the long run pain equals no gain, and in fact loss.

COMPETITION

How could one compete in competitive sports practicing this approach to athletics? The answer is that the truly great athletes find a way into the zone and from that state of optimum performance produce amazing feats of athleticism. I once heard a football player prior to the Superbowl talking about being in the zone. He described a time in which he was moving incredibly fast but everything seemed to slow down. He could see everything happening on the entire field and as well his movements were effortless. This is what we look for from exercise. Any approach that requires strain and force is destructive to physiology.

EXERCISE RECOMMENDATIONS SPECIFIC TO VATA, PITTA AND KAPHA CONSTITUTIONS

Vatas like movement but they are seldom built for rigor though some run marathons. Among the sports suitable for them are Ping pong; badminton; dance: any sport that is not arduous in the sense of being a contact sport but will satisfy their need for quickness.

Pittas are often aggressive and strong, and their focus is often on winning. Solo sports particularly those that are preformed in cool temperatures such as competitive skiing will appeal to those with Pitta constitution. Often Pitta may be a leader and team organizer. Any NFL quarterback will have a high pitta component.

Though Kapha may have great endurance and strength they may often be slow to get started. (As an extreme example of this I saw an Olympic weight lifter's coach slapping the lifter's face to get him fired up!) All the rigorous sports may be suitable for Kapha.

The refrain in this Session on Vedic Exercise is the same as that of any other Session: Each of us is unique. Find the sport(s) that best suits your physiology.

SESSION WRAP-UP

FOCUS FOR THE WEEK

- Begin exercising by walking.
- Get into the zone and feel the effortlessness and joy of proper exercise.
- Ruminate on the idea of 'do less and accomplish more'.

EDITORIAL RANT

The destructive way we exercise in the West is expressive of our lack of feelings for, and lack of understanding of human physiology. It is unspeakable what is done to our youth in the name of exercise. Tragic is an inadequate word to describe the situation. The resultant toxicity forced into the joints and tissues ultimately diminishes millions of lives.

Regardless of the plight of our youth and professional athletes you and I personally have a great opportunity to begin a satisfying and safe fitness program. While in the past, poor preparation may have been part of the reason for shattered good intentions and abandoned promises today you are well prepared to succeed. Congratulations and good luck.

AGING REVERSAL

- The purpose of exercise is to release stress and toxins, and even more important, to re-create the physiology.

- The body will eventually revolt from an exercise program that places an excess of strain on it.
- The key to enjoyment and the success in an exercise program is to routinely perform from a settled, well oxygenated level.
- Vedic Exercise nurtures the body and yet is capable of producing peak performance.

FURTHER READING

Dr. John Doulliard is a key exponent of Vedic Exercise. See *Reading and Websites*

FURTHER WRITING

Remember and record an instance where exercise felt effortless and you wanted to keep going forever. This will create 'happy' chemicals in your physiology.

***

We have spent time in the lush valleys of Ayurvedic thought and now in *Session 11: Life* we will begin to explore the lofty peaks of aging reversal. The most powerful ideas are yet to come.

Session 11
Life

MOTHER NATURE

In my not so humble opinion we need to spend more time talking with each other, and particularly with our children, about this miracle we call Life.

One morning while I was weeding the garden I tossed the pulled weeds betweens the rows. The next morning after a night of rain their roots had begun burrowing into the soil and the weed tops had lifted off the earth striving for sunlight. Though the weeds had been rudely torn from the earth they still wanted to live. They wanted Life. How can weeds 'want to live'? Or was it the Life within the weeds that wanted to continue to live?

We all remember the grade school science experiment where we planted bulbs upside down. The roots would sprout out of the top of the bulb and would grow downwards, and the stem sprouted out of the bottom of the bulb and grew upwards towards the sunlight. Very clearly plants have intelligence.

In time of natural disaster we blame Mother Nature and seem to equate Her with destruction. This is usually the extent of our reference to Her. Sadly our culture puts too much focus on Nature as death and destruction. Nature is miraculous in its complexity and function. (Our attention, as we have seen throughout the course, enlivens. Our attention on Life enlivens Life and our attention on dark side of Life enlivens that aspect of Life.)

EXPERIMENTS

If you wish to take time for an experiment you will need a lemon or lime. Cut the fruit in half and put the halves together held by a rubber band. 24 hours later remove the rubber band and pull the pieces of fruit apart. It is almost creepy how the fruit has tried to grow back together.

Another experiment is to stand a mango on end and slice along the flat side of the seed removing one half of the fruit. Wrap the 2 pieces individually and put them in separate locations in the fridge. Taste them the next day.

The one **without** the seed tastes sweet and appetizing. The one with the seed attached tastes repugnant. What has happened? The seed has 'instructed' the attached fruit to rot so that the seed will have fertilizer when it sprouts. The half without the seed—without the instruction manual—remains fresh. Had the fruit not been damaged it would have remained sweet and fresh in the fridge where the proper conditions for sprouting don't exist. Plants have intelligence. Plants have Life. And the food we eat (real food, not Twinkes and the like) has Life.

ANOTHER EXAMPLE OF LIFE IN PLANTS

Preparing to cook chard I removed the leaf from each side of the stalks and put the stalks in the compost bucket. The next morning the bases of the stalks had curved down into the water and the stalks, looking much like macabre vegetable skeletons, had curved upright to the light. They wanted fiercely to live even though there was little chance of them doing so.

LIFE

In the Eastern Cultures and the 'Primitive Cultures' everything is seen to have Life or to be Life—and Life is revered. In our culture the Life of things is seldom acknowledged and many of us despise anything other than what is viewed to be the 'me' or the 'I'.

The ancients understood Life. Consider the words 'respire', 'inspire', 'expire'. The root word 'spir' is the same root as the root in spirit or breath. As a culture we need to put our attention on Life—Life with a capital L. Other than the word life which we seldom use in this context we don't even have a word for Life—such as 'Prana' a word for spirit from India, or 'Chi' a word for Life from China.

Do we have such an invocation as in this Eastern prayer?

I revere the great Goddess Lakshmi who is present as Life in all living thing.

Clearly the thought from this prayer is that there exists a Life 'substance'.

Life is in each of us. Some people are charismatic: bristling with vitality and shining with energy. We are attracted to these special people: we want to be seen with them, to touch them, and perhaps to jump into bed with them. And though many people look like zombies each person must have some amount of Life, otherwise they would be dead.[35]

OJAS

A concept discussed earlier (See **Session 4: Youthfulness.**) is that within physiology is a store of Life. To remain young we need to constantly replenish this Life. Though we do have 'a quantity of Life' at birth it is not something to be consumed like a car consumes a tank of gas.

What a freeing, uplifting idea that it is possible to replenish our supply of Life.

Though an imbalance may consume or destroys Life, nevertheless at some level, always, each of us want Life—vibrant, glowing, zestful Life. How to have more Life is a question that is being answered throughout *The Aging Reversal Course.* Now, and in the next sessions, we turn our attention to more powerful means, (many of them known throughout the ages), to infuse our physiology with Life.

THE SATVIC LIFE

Though Life is found everywhere we can choose to embrace a Satvic life. That is to say we can cultivate a life of purity. Our water, our air, our food, should be pure. Our environment, our homes, our place of work, our gardens and land should be pure.

Think of special places in the world: Machu Piccu, Hawaii, The Greek Islands, and Vancouver Island. Think of temples or other similar spaces filled with peace. We should surround ourselves with the same Life that permeates the air of these holy places.

Consider too the entertainment we choose; the products we purchase; our thoughts; our emotions; the people around us. We may choose to have a Satvic life. We may make the intent that everything in our life radiates purity and health.

The Behaviorial Rasayanas included earlier in *The Aging Reversal Course* are relevant here again, particularly as the spontaneous practice of them indicates a Satvic life. (How is the incorporation of these behaviors into your life proceeding? It is not too late–if you haven't already—to team up with a partner for the remainder of the course.)

- Avoid anger. Find a way to recognize the first signs of anger and to deal with it by putting the attention on it before it erupts. This means to mitigate and dissolve or evaporate the anger—not to repress it. Human physiology's ability to experience anger is not an accident.
- Don't over use the senses. To be discussed in **Session 13**
- Remain calm. Breathe deeply through the nose. **Session 1**
- Stay cool, i.e. not overly warm.
- Cleanliness of body and environment effects our emotions and thoughts.
- Give. Work not primarily to get money but to give the service to humanity that you are best suited to give.
- Be respectful.
- Be loving.
- Speak the truth.
- Speak and think well of others.
- Maintain an orderly lifestyle.
- Be guileless. (Do many of these qualities remind you of Mahati Ghandi's approach to life?)
- Avoid fools: associate with the wise. (Desiderata)
- Be positive: be optimistic.

- Follow your cultural traditions—including religious injunctions.
- Focus on spiritual progress.
- Be yourself.
- Attend to Silence
- Respect and care for yourself.

Record in your *I R Healthy* Notebook the number of times you spontaneously practiced any of these Rasayanas in the last week. Were these instances spontaneous, or did you institute them from an intellectual level? (Practicing the Rasayanas from any level is much better than not practicing them at all.)

MEAT: TO EAT, OR NOT TO EAT MEAT

Eating, breathing and consuming water are great opportunities to infuse Life into the body. Food too has Life, but meat which we think of as food is dead—it has no life. Nonetheless for many individuals it is difficult to maintain proper nutrition without eating meat. Meat is also popular as it is extremely difficult for vegetarians to satisfy each of the six tastes and assimilate adequate nutrients—unless their diet includes appropriate use of spices. Also, another characteristic which partly explains popularity of meat, particularly for individuals with inadequate digestive fire, is that meat when first eaten produces a heating effect.[36]

If you eat meat, and you probably should occasionally eat small portions until your digestion is super efficient, then sprinkle your spice mix on the meat while it is cooking. (Earlier we discussed how spices, and both fat and water, carry nutrients through the cell walls. Cooking meat in a stew is most effective way to render it digestible.)

- Beef, fish, mutton, pork reduces Vata, increases Pitta and Kapha
- Rabbit increases Vata, decreases Pitta and Kapha
- Beef, which is sweet and appealing to Pitta, turns sour during digestion. Sour is the most aggravating taste for Pitta. (Was there ever a cattle rancher who didn't look like he had a pickle up his backside?)
- Chicken in moderation for Vata, Pitta and Kapha.
- Meat is hard to digest. Eat small amounts. Most human digestive systems are not able to properly digest large amounts of meat. The resulting poor digestion creates much ill health. [37]
- The 6 billion folks on our planet consume megatons of meat each day, the production of which causes immense strain on our earth.
- Animals have Life—they are Life and we destroy Life, usually in a most cruel manner. The chemicals the animals produce within their bodies while standing in line waiting to be slaughtered and while being killed, are nothing short of poison for those who consume the meat.
- In addition, millions of human beings spend most of their waking hours creating toxicity within themselves as they cruelly slaughter animals.

Nonetheless, Ayurvedic texts, (I have heard) list fifty plus types of birds suitable for eating, complete with recipes. Beef and pork, needed by some rare individuals, are included in the texts with recommended suitable spices and recipes.

Vegetarianism has been touted in the West by individuals trained in reclusive, monastic traditions. Vegetarian diets along with reclusive meditation practices and other austerities are seldom suitable for most householders—particularly people working outside at 20 below zero. Caveat Emptor re vegetarianism! (See **Session 16: The Trouble with the East**.)

KEYS TO ENERGY

Be aware that Life is everywhere. Air and water and food have Life. The ocean, forests and earth have Life. Everything has Life.

THE FIRST KEY TO ENERGIZING: RELEASING THE OLD ENERGY.

Abhyanga is good for the skin and for pacifying Vata dosha but there is a far greater benefit. As discussed below there are 108 Marmas within the body which are junction points of energy and intelligence. [38] Abhyanga nourishes each of the Marmas through touch but even more effectively through our attention, as we apply the warm, often herbalized oil. **Our attention infuses Life into the Marmas.**

New energy won't be able to move around to be 'absorbed' if the Marmas that release the stale, used up energy are blocked. This stale energy must be released. How do we remove this 'dead' energy from the physiology? The answer is proper respiration, proper exercise, and Abhyanga with particular attention to the hands and feet. (As mentioned earlier the hands and feet may be briefly massaged with herbalized oils prior to sleep.) As well as promoting a sound sleep the attention on these four Marmas (one Marma on each of the hands and feet) enliven them and support their primary function as major centers for releasing impurities.

THE SECOND KEY: MOVEMENT OF ENERGY

In addition to the stale energy being released, the channels that the energy flows through should be clear so that the energy—Life—can flow freely to where it needs to go. (Plaque in the arteries would be one example of the many types of clogged channels). Proper breathing, exercise, hydration, proper diet, Pancha Karma help keep the channels, as well as the Marmas clear.

THE THIRD KEY: BRINGING ENERGY INTO THE BODY

Proper oxygenation, particularly the practice of Pranayama in the fresh, energized early morning air infuses Prana—Life—into the physiology. The benefits of Pranayama are several: such as connecting the left and right sides of the brain, and cleaning the channels between the left and right side of the brain. A qualified Yoga instructor can teach this breathing technique. [39]

Proper air and water and food each well ingested will result in the infusion of their Life into our physiology.

Swimming, resting on the earth, walking in a forest, walking on a beach, walking in the cool of the evening under the moon and stars, looking at the stars, watching a sunrise or sunset, the uplifting thoughts resulting from experiencing art, music, poetry etc, love for our self and others (who are not really others) each fill us with Life.

THREE KEY LIFE SYSTEMS

There are three main Life Systems within our physiology that also govern the Universe's three main 'impulses' within physiology: creation, preservation and dissolution. These systems—Marut, Agni, and Soma—are responsible for the flow, infusion, and the 'release' of Life—are well known in Vedic thought. While Chinese Medicine understands Agni and Soma to some degree as Yang and Yin it seems to lack the concept of Marut. Marut moves. Angi heats. Soma cools, stabilizes, nourishes and supports. Do these concepts sound familiar? I'm sure they do. Marut's movement is akin to Vata; Agni—heat is akin to Pitta; Soma—fluidity and structure is akin to Kapha. If any of the three major marmas or their sub marmas are out of balance the physiology will have a corresponding imbalance.

Each of Marut, Agni, and Soma are connected to one of the Mahamarmas. (Maha translated in this case as key, or dominant marmas.)

MARMAS

The three Mahamarmas are each 'responsible' for 35 'lesser' Marmas resulting in a total of 108. These 108 systems are the silent processes that automatically govern human physiology. We cannot micromanage these systems but we may give them attention and support. Each of the practices you have learned in **The Aging Reversal Course** is designed to support these 108 systems.

This said, Marmas are simply junction points of energy and intelligence in physiology. For example the area including the solar plexus is a Marma Point—a juncture of nerves and numerous other channels of intelligence. During the Cobra yoga posture one lays face down and then arches the back by pushing up with the arms, raising the chest, shoulders and head, to 'stretch' the area of the solar plexus thereby drawing one's attention to this center and enlivening the flow of energy and intelligence. Yes it is true that yoga postures may keep one limber but that is a small part of what they are designed to do.

It is beyond the scope of **The Aging Reversal Course** to teach the 108 Marmas and the various aspects of physiology they 'govern' and/or 'fuel'. You can nevertheless enliven them in numerous ways (for example with your attention while practicing Vedic Exercise) and yet not need to know their specific functions.[40] During practice of both the Yoga Postures and The Sun Salutation, or nearly any exercise or activity let the attention be spontaneously drawn to focus easily on the area that draws your attention. Attention, as we have heard often throughout the course, enlivens and heals. The enlivenment of the Marmas and their connecting channels is a most beneficial result of proper practice of a properly designed set of Yoga Postures and Vedic Exercise.

Are the Marma points the same location as the main acupuncture points? Some Vaidyas claim that much of Chinese Traditional Medicine came across the Himalayas. I don't know if this is true though some of the similarities are striking. If the Marmas are located in the same place as the acupuncture points—and often they are one and the same—it suddenly seems remarkably fortunate to have an array of herbalized creams (See **Reading and Websites** Vaidya Mishra's website) available to be applied to these points instead of having to stick needles into or assault the marmas with electricity.

Also you may know, or be interested to know, that Tai Chi has a set of 108 postures which reportedly and very likely do, enliven the 108 Marmas.

Marmas act much like a switch to let energy flow to the various parts of the body. Each of the major organs—lungs, liver, pancreas, stomach etc. etc—has a corresponding Marma. Ayurveda and western science know that there are 30 gaps between the vertebra and from each gap there is a nerve to one of the major organs. Heart problems? Hip problems? Spleen problems? Prior to replacing a heart or a hip check the 'light switch' and see if the heart or the hip is getting a proper flow of Life. Often in the case of a heart transplant a second transplant is needed 8 or 10 years later. It would be wise before replacing any organ to first check the 'switch' and determine if the energy flow has been lessened (much analogous to a light bulb being dimmed by a dimmer switch) and to clear the channels rather than popping in a replacement part.

Considering the immense amount of human suffering and out of control disease costs it seems that a close look at the Ayurvedic understanding of 'turning on the light switches' would be a very prudent idea.

SESSION WRAP-UP

FOCUS FOR THE WEEK

Be aware of the huge variety of enjoyable means of infusing Life into your physiology.

EDITORIAL RANT

The lack of understanding of Life contributes to the Life hating destruction that is on the verge of destroying the planet. With similar hatred individuals are destroying themselves and calling it aging.

Aging Reversal

- Life is all around us and is able to be infused into our physiology.
- All that we have learned in **The Aging Reversal Course** is designed to nurture the 108 systems that 'handle' the flow of Life.
- All we do in daily life should support and infuse Life within us.
- Aging reversal is simple: as the channels and Marmas are purified more energy is able to flow through these junctures to repair and rebuild the various aspects of physiology and promote youthfulness.

Further Reading

The understanding that Life is available everywhere and able to be replenished is not a concept I have often come across. If you can direct me to a discussion about Life I would like to know of it. Jesus certainly understood Life. (See also Maharishi Mahesh, *The Science of Being, and the Art of Living* in the **Reading and Websites**.) Destruction on the other hand is discussed endlessly. Why the large focus on destruction? There is no pretty answer to this question that I can think of.

Further Writing

Describe an example of Life struggling to continue living.

***

Session 12: The Gap is a most interesting session; the insights are as far reaching as any we have yet seen in the course. Marmas are gaps: they are neither the channels that feed into them nor the channels that stem out from them but something different than either.

Session 12

The Gap

NOTHING AND EVERYTHING

It seems safe to say that between one thing and another there is a third 'something'. How can there not be something between two? The concept of the 'gap' is well understood in Eastern Culture. Chinese paintings, often taller than wide, and childlike, (ie spontaneous in technique), puzzled me for years. I couldn't understand their appeal. The mountains and trees and birds didn't look particularly beautiful. The beauty, it turns out, is the beauty of the space between the figures—the shape of the space in between, for example, a mountain and a tree. In the West photography understands this concept of creating a pleasing space between objects.

Though Westerners as a culture are vaguely aware of the gap [41] at best we may hear some mumbling about the 'void' and shiver.

In the East children are taught about the gap from an early age. I read a story from a children's book from India years ago and was stunned by the theme. Let me summarize.

A King is beset with a demon and calls in healers from far and wide to cure him. The demon's fangs are sunk deep into the King's neck and are slowly sucking the Life from his body. (Note the concept of Life as a sub-

stance and the metaphor that some impure and drain-ing influence can diminish the supply of Life within us.) One by one the healers view the demon and report that there is no cure for the ghastly parasite. In frustra-tion and desperation the King summons the most iras-cible and cantankerous of all the healers. The old man grudgingly comes to the King's court, examines the King and the Demon, and announces that the malady may be cured. The King and his court are overjoyed. Then the old healer adds a puzzling condition: 'But not in the day, nor at night'.

The King and the court are outraged.

The sage replies: 'There is a time that is neither day nor night. When you know this time of which I speak, you will be able to banish the Demon—but not until.'

Through this fable the concept of the gap is intro-duced to children—an idea our culture shudders to talk about.

Have you experienced a special time that is neither day nor night—during sunrise or sunset? Or the calm be-fore a storm that is neither the beautiful day nor the storm but instead is the gap between the two. Or the sound just before water boils. There is an odd silence just before wa-ter begins to bubble. (Stop reading, boil water and listen to the time just before it begins to boil. Neat eh?) There is always a gap: A gap between musical notes; a gap be-tween words; a gap between two trees; between tastes. Between two 'somethings' there has to be something else that is neither.

Our culture particularly, and most of the planet, are terrified of the gap. Our music, our eating, all our sensory experiences, are designed to preclude the gap. Madonna and the rest of pop culture provides the music we demand, but as a culture we are lost to reality and to pleasure (yes Madonna to pleasure) until we understand the gap.

How important is the gap to Life and living? Consider this poem from 9th century China about a quite dramatic, but I think not unusual, experience of the gap.

Sleeping on Horseback

> We had ridden long and were still far from the inn;
> My eyes grew dim; for a moment I fell asleep.
> Under my right arm the whip still dangled;
> In my left hand the reins for an instant slackened.
> Suddenly I awoke and turned to question my groom.
> "We have gone one hundred paces since you fell asleep."
> Body and spirit had for a time changed places;
> Swift and slow had turned to their contraries.
> For these few steps that my horse had carried me
> Had taken in my dream countless ages of time!
> True indeed is that saying of Wise Men
> "A hundred years are but a moment of sleep."
> **Po Chu-i**

The poet is in awe of this ability of human physiology to transcend time. What is not mentioned is the experience of a grand influx of energy—of Life—that usually accompanies this experience of the gap.

Athletes, artists, people from all areas of life know of the gap and we would do well as a culture to begin talking about it and giving it the important role it can play in our well being.

A FOURTH STATE OF CONSCIOUSNESS: THE KEY TO DISSOLVING TRAUMA.

The characteristics of waking, sleeping and dreaming states of consciousness are common knowledge. Western Science understands their unique physiological correlates. What the East brings to the discussion is the monumental concept that between any two of these states of consciousness there must be, no matter how infinitesimal, a point that is neither of the state of consciousness on either side of it. In some instances, for some individuals, this 'space' may seem large in terms of time as in the poem above.

There is a gap between sleep and waking—waking and sleep; sleep and dreaming—dreaming and sleep and so forth. The gap must have different qualities than the consciousness on either side of it. (If it has the same qualities as the consciousness on either side of it then it would be that consciousness.) Most important it will have, as do the other three states of consciousness, its own unique physiological correlates. The consciousness must have uniqueness if it is truly a state of consciousness.

Consider the physiology of both waking and sleeping states of consciousness. Generally, when awake, the mind is alert and the body is likely working at high speed. While sleeping our mind is dull and our physiology is resting and operating at a slow rate. Dreaming too has its own physiology. The physiology of the 4th state is unique and in addition, as beneficial and **necessary**, as the other states of consciousness.

In the early 70's Maharishi Mahesh explained this concept of a fourth state of consciousness and its unique physiological correlates to physiologist Dr. Keith Wallace.

He suggested that if Dr. Wallace would check the physiology of individuals while they were meditating the physiological correlates of this unique state of consciousness would be present. (See **Reading and Websites** Wallace) What Wallace found about transcendental consciousness (transcend: to go beyond) was that the physiology of it was unique in that the mind was very alert and the body very rested: a quite unusual and indeed unique pairing of physiological indices.

One might imagine that the discovery of a fourth state of consciousness would create quite a stir in academic circles. Also one might think popular culture would be gaga with it—tee shirts reading "morph into the fourth" etc. One might expect an expression such as "venture forth into the 4th" to catch on and sweep through the culture with similar success as for instance the saying "no pain no gain." But what do we hear of this monumental, 30 year old discovery? Nada; not a peep.

Of course the opportunity to experience Transcendental Consciousness is not limited to meditation although meditating briefly twice a day appears to be a grand opportunity to bring the effects of this consciousness into one's life. (See www.tm.org or Dossey in the **Reading and Websites,** or see research by Herbert Benson) In addition to the possibility of experiencing this 4th state of consciousness during meditation (and having its qualities infused into the physiology) there are anecdotal reports of it prior to sleep and prior to waking. Dickens reportedly plotted his novels in a heightened state of awareness prior to sleep. But in fact TC can be experienced anywhere there is a gap. Between any two sensual experiences: between musical notes; between tastes of food; between emotions; or between thoughts. Anywhere there is the experience of two things there is something between the two. (See Tolle, <u>The Power of Now</u>) Though Eckhart Tolle may not come right out and say so the Gap is part of what he knows and experiences but with him it appears it is always present.

Have you had this experience of an alert mind and at the same time a slowed physiology? I have spoken with numerous individuals who uniformly have a memory of an experience where their mind was incredibly alert and the body was nearly still. Consider this excerpt from Wordsworth's poem:

Lines Composed a Few Miles Above Tintern Abbey

That blessed mood,
In which the burthen of the mystery,
In which the heavy and the weary weight
Of all this unintelligible world,
Is lightened:—that serene and blessed Mood,
In which the affections gently lead us on,
Until, the breath of this corporeal frame
And even the motion of our human blood
Almost suspended, we are laid asleep
In body, and become a living soul:
While with an eye made quiet by the power
Of harmony, and the deep power of joy,
We see into the life of things.
William Wordsworth

Is it possible to be 'laid asleep in body, and become a living soul: to see into the Life of things.'? Is this poem a fantasy? Not in the least. The poet is reporting on a profound experience available through human physiology—a normal experience that human physiology is regularly capable of experiencing. Saints and poets and seers have been reporting these experiences throughout time. Read St. Paul, St Augustine, or nearly any of the Saints: or read poetry: Whitman and Blake particularly. The same experience of TC is spoken of with awe and often with glee.

While in class teaching this course a student asked: "You mean a state of altered consciousness?" I answered, "No, I mean a normal state of consciousness." I mean a normal, usual state of dynamic alertness and deep rest where LIFE in infused into our physiology."

Transcending is something all the members of the world family would do well to find a way to have happen each and every day. As did Wordsworth or St. Paul, any person may have a profound experience of the 4th state of consciousness. Profound in that takes our breath away and fills us with Life. I hardly meet anyone who hasn't had a clear experience of this special consciousness. But as a culture—through some fear or another—we seldom talk about these experiences. [42]

Experiencing this normal state of consciousness is a key opportunity for Prana, Chi, Spirit, (call Life what you will) to be infused into the physiology. This experience is as essential to living as water and food and air. To experience the benefits of an additional state of consciousness—to imbibe the characteristics of this consciousness into physiology—is a grand opportunity for a richer life. **To not make use of this capacity would be the height of folly.**

Recall how it feels to wake up after sleep, particularly in the Kapha time of day. The qualities of sleep consciousness pervade our physiology. How does it feel to wake up from a dream? How do we feel after a busy day at the office? We need to wind down. The point is that consciousness 'rubs off on' or 'colors' our physiology. In the same fashion Transcendental Consciousness 'colors' our physiology. **We come away from it with an expansive, alert, yet settled and rejuvenated state of physiology**.

SESSION WRAP-UP

FOCUS FOR THE WEEK

Be open to opportunities to experience the gap. They are everywhere.

EDITORIAL RANT

Experiencing the fourth state of consciousness is necessary for human physiology to thrive. We can limp along without this infusion of Life much in the same manner as we can choose to breathe only through the mouth and use a small percentage of our breathing capacity, or we can embrace the full potential of our physiology. For people who are ill and suffering I suggest you bring more of Transcendental Consciousness into your life. It is easy to whine about design flaws and genetics, and to avoid accepting the full capacity of human physiology to heal.

For those of you who are vibrant there will be no reluctance. Where can I get more of what I already have will be the question.

To the healers whose profession it is to heal the suffering people of the earth you are engaged in a losing battle until you introduce Transcendental Consciousness—that is Life—as the basis for healing.

AGING REVERSAL

- As a culture our focus is too often on death rather than Life.
- And we have lost sight of the use and power of the Gap.

FURTHER READING

Satya Yuga Chronicles: *Before the Dawn*. Author Paul Colver. www.paulcolver.info

FURTHER WRITING

Recount an experience of the gap. What was the result of the experience in terms of your physiology? Did time slow down as in the Chinese poem? Were you energized yet rested? Keep in mind that the experience can take a billion different forms: it is the change in physiology that is the constant.

***

This discussion of the Gap continues in **Session 13: The Purpose of Sensuality**.

Session 13
The Purpose of Sensuality

SENSUALITY IN THE DARK AGES

Regardless of the misinformation we may have absorbed in our youth; regardless of the pronouncements of the Church Fathers at the Council of Nicosia a proper understanding of sensuality is of very great importance to our well being. Where would we be without sensuality? Without sensuality how could there be the Gap? And with no gap what then?

It is easy to understand how an authoritarian group mired in the ignorance of a Dark Age could misunderstand, and wish to ban, sensuality. They no doubt understood that sensuality consumes energy and when misused and overused draws attention away from Life. Given the era in which they lived and given the 'science' of those times the conclusions they drew should scarcely cause us to wonder. But what is our excuse for the improper use of sensuality? In our revolt against traditions that stifled sensuality modern culture has become lost to excessive and destructive sensuality. How can we accept such foolish, Life destroying conclusions?

What to do? What to do?

William Blake has something to say regarding sensuality:

He Who Binds to Himself:
He who binds to himself a Joy
Doth the winged life destroy;
But he who kisses the Joy as it flies
Lives in Eternity's sunrise.
William Blake

(Do you imagine that Blake might have been giggling euphorically as he wrote this poem?)

Primarily the poem is crafted to convey the joyful emotion one feels upon discovering one of Life's secrets. Rather than to instruct, the poet wants to share his joy. Nonetheless, let us do what is all too often done with poetry and coarsen our reaction to this beautiful poem by trying to discern, much as though reading an essay, what Blake trying 'to tell us'?

To paraphrase the first couplet: *to grasp at joy, to try to hold on to joy, destroys 'the winged life'.*

To paraphrase the second couplet: *But she who enjoys the joy as it comes, and doesn't try to hang on to joy, but who attends to Joy* (kisses the Joy: note the capital J) *then that person lives in Eternity's sunrise.* ('Eternity's sunrise', note Eternity is capitalized.)

I can't imagine how the notion expressed in this first couplet might be conveyed more simply. Attachment to pleasure destroys Life. Binding one's self to a sensation—trying to hold on to a sensation—destroys Life.

The second couplet is equally pithy. Give brief joy appropriate, brief attention. Enjoy the Gap (the joy) that follows sensual experience but don't get wrapped up in the sensual experience, and don't try to prolong it or to prolong the joy that results from it.

The Gap feeds us with energy—when we don't try to force it and just allow it happen. This is one of the great secrets of Life. Sensuality, as is generally understood and experienced, takes our energy and ages us whereas the innocent experiencing of the Gap fills us with Life.

Blake instructs that we innocently enjoy what IS before we charge forward trying to generate more sensual experience. He doesn't denigrate Joy. (note that the word is capitalized). For Blake, fully and easily attending to the winged joy until it has dissipated—but not trying to prolong it—is the most Life supporting approach to sensuality.

FLEETING PLEASURE

Our culture has become trapped in the notion that sensual experience is the end all and be all of life. Commonly we hear the whine that pleasure is too brief and fleeting; we often hear a refrain of 'Poor me, pleasure is gone so quickly.'

How humorous! Imagine tasting the first strawberry of spring (or imagine any fabulous taste). We crush the berry on our tongue and the taste 'floods' our mouth with exquisite sensation. Pleasure fills our physiology and 'overwhelms' us. 'We are lost' in the taste. (Who is the 'we' and what is the meaning of 'lost'?) This flood of pleasure is brief but how fortunate that it is brief. How would it be that if for the following days or weeks we were stumbling around lost in pleasure? 'Oh, excuse me for bumping into you. I ate a strawberry a few weeks ago, mmmmm etc. Or 'No officer

I didn't see the red light. Well you see I ate a strawberry a few weeks ago and…'

Sensuality is fabulous. But it is not the be all and end all our popular culture makes it out to be. This is not to say that for some individuals a Dionysian or Tantric approach to life might not be of some use. (See **Reading and Websites**: Margo Anand) But generally speaking overuse of sensuality stresses the physiology—particularly if we do not experience the silence that follows the experience, and precedes the next experience.

The Gap as Blake indicates energizes us—we live in 'Eternity's sunrise'. Note Blake's use of the word in Eternity. It is the same eternity our Chinese poet speaks of.

Life enters our body through water and food and air, but how much more so through the Gap created between swallows, mouthfuls or breaths? The silence of the Gap, what we find between sensual experiences, is NOW. We focus intimately and briefly on experience and the sensation dissolves into the NOW. We taste the strawberry and then the taste "is gone", what remains? Nothing—Everything. And we enjoy Everything until the experience of It is overshadowed. We think that the taste makes us feel good but it is the energy of the gap beyond the taste that fuels us. The taste is necessary but the energizing comes from the gap.

I think the misunderstanding of the Church Fathers is that they thought if one could eliminate the sensuality (the experience) there would be more Gap. They may have thought that sensuality hid the Gap which is what happens when one rushes off to the next experience. While the notion of avoiding sensuality seemed sensible to them it is simply an inaccurate understanding of the workings of human physiology.

To See the World in a Grain of Sand:
To see the world in a grain of sand
And a heaven in a wild flower.
Hold infinity in the palm of your hand
And eternity in an hour.
William Blake

Eternity is again the focus: the joy of expanded awareness is beautifully conveyed. Are the best experiences available to human physiology to be generating by skiing down Mt. Everest? Do we really need to scuba dive among a school of sharks to experience human physiology at its fullest? "Go Big or Go Home." is an expression that gained popularity as quickly as "No Pain, No Gain." What is the matter with our culture? Our billboards and advertisements scream out that sensuality is the highest and best use of our body. That a heart beating at 200 beats a minute is the best we can feel. We brainwash our children with this nonsense and it has become our main export to the world. As a culture we have convinced ourselves that the body is bad; that the flesh is evil; the root of all problems. That the body is something divorced from us: something other than us, something that holds us back from all that we could be. That if we punish the body severely enough it will perform at its peak potential. A triathlon or scaling Mt. Everest in a couple of non-stop days is really what will make us feel good. Ayurveda calmly says 'Do less and accomplish more.'

Blake and anyone like him, according to the thinking of our culture is a fool babbling nonsense. Where in our culture is the awe and reverence for the miracle that is our body? Simply the considering of the innumerable things it does to keep us well is evidence enough of the majesty of the physical. Consider for example how the body heals a broken bone. The body's intelligence turns the ends of broken bone into a putty and anesthetizes the area so that the bone may be set. This process takes a bit of time so in Chinese Medicine the bone is stabilized and then set a few days later. The body is a miracle yet it is generally thought to be the problem. [43]

The problem is not the gift of sensuality but the mis-use of sensuality which saps our energy and ages us. Who among us hasn't at some time treated themselves poorly: aged beef, alcohol or other drugs, horror movies? Torture movies? Overwork and over stimulation of the senses? We need to accept 'ownership' for our situation as a result of our past actions but also to recognize that we are currently building our future health. [44] Similarly, in order to heal the earth we need to quit blaming the problems of the world on the devil and accept that collectively we have created the world, and collectively we will create a new world.

FORGIVENESS

Whatever has happened or not happen in your life forgive yourself. While we need to own what we have done (and are currently doing to ourselves) we need to recall that today we are not the person that did whatever damage we did years ago—or even yesterday. We are working to correct the imbalances resulting from past actions, and we are working through **The Aging Reversal Course** in order to increase our understanding of how to create balance and move forward.

SESSION WRAP-UP

Focus for the Week
- Enjoy experiencing a sensation but observe what happens as the sensation dissolves into 'nothing/everything'.
- Wait for the next sensation to arise as it surely will.
- Notice how trying to hang on to sensuality dissipates energy.

Editorial Rant
St. Augustine and St Paul and every major religion's condemnation of 'the flesh' are just nonsense out of the Dark Ages. The idea that the flesh is the enemy would be humorous if the results of it weren't so destructive. Sensuality is the greatest of gifts: where would we be without it?

Aging Reversal
- Misuse and overuse of sensuality results in aging.
- Focusing lightly on the gap, after the sensation has dissolved, infuses physiology with energy.
- Trying to hang on to sensuality dissipates energy.

Further Reading
I haven't seen these concepts even touched on elsewhere. Blake particularly understood sensuality as do many other poets: Walt Whitman for example.

FURTHER WRITING

Describe a time when you were highly energized by sensuality. Was it in fact the time spent between the sensations in the Gap that resulted in the energy? If you are at a loss for such experiences then share a mango among the group.

***

Session 14: The Millstone makes clear another little understood and useful capability of human physiology.

Session 14
Casting off the Millstones

WESTERN CULTURE UNSTUCK

Over the last few decades in the West the understanding that youthfulness may be reestablished has been gradually gaining a foothold. The problem is that most of the approaches to recreating health (even among many 'New Age' healers) are based on the outdated science which views the body as a machine put together much like a clock. The approach resulting from this misguided understanding is to fiddle with the specifics: the pancreas, or the lymphatic system, or cranial—sacral healing, or chelation, or something else- usually with a catchy name. Dealing with the parts may in some cases be necessary but without an understanding of the synergy within human physiology these healing approaches are just more of the same old, same old.

To compound the problem there is the misunderstanding of energy. New Age healers often delude themselves into believing they have the supply of Life energy of a healing saint and stress and tire themselves by 'pouring' their energy into their clients. A person drained of Life can have little hope of healing anyone else.

Paul Colver

From Ayurveda, and Quantum Physics, there comes the understanding that the wholeness within us needs attention—Attention with a capitol A. To be truly healthy is to learn to care for the Life within. Recent understandings of Quantum Physics make clear the case of a synergy within the body, (as well as a synergy within the family of man, and indeed the entire universe). Our role as individuals is to nurture and strengthen this synergy. Our role as healers is to teach individuals how to access and make most efficient use of this synergy to nurture and strengthen their own physiology.

We need to make a change from fixing the parts to a new approach of enlivening the synergy. This Chinese expression sums up the needs of our time quite well:

'If we don't change directions we are likely to find ourselves exactly where we are headed.'

Let me rephrase this:

If we don't change from the direction of fiddling with the parts, and instead learn to nurture the whole we will continue to find ourselves exactly where we are headed—which is exactly where we are: amidst a health care crisis of unnecessary suffering and expense.

Though it is easy to argue a doom and gloom portrait of the available approaches to health care there are numerous glimmers of hope such as the upsurge of interest in Indigenous Medicine, Chinese Medicine, Ayurveda and energy healing modalities. Our culture, blessed by the freedom to experiment and with an openness to new ideas, is hopefully on the way to a well thought out leap forward in our approach to wellness (and the wellness of our earth, and the universe).

And the advent of these understandings is happening not a moment too soon. The despicable state of our collective health, and our world, is in large measure the results of collective beliefs that we can create health by fiddling with the parts, and that energy—Life—is limited or not to be considered in the equation. Currently millions are suffering poor health, often beginning at a very early age, but the only happy news in this is that the mess we have created drives us collectively, through self interest, to find solutions. As the population of the world ages there can only be more urgency to find satisfactory means for creating health. Our attempts to generate health on the basis of an array of misguided notions regarding human physiology will simply not produce the results we need and deserve.

A MILLSTONE DISSOLVES

From **Session 3** we recall that our physiology is designed to 'throw off' the effects of stress and repair itself. This process is continuous. For example, we may feel 'terrible' before sleeping yet awake the next morning feeling as though a great weight has lifted. We may think, *How great to be alive!* We are blissful and energetic. What inevitably happens? The body doing what it does so well will begin to throw off more strain: we will likely feel terrible again. The euphoria and bliss evaporate. And then what happens? Eventually we feel as though a 'great weight' is lifted and again we are on top of the world so to speak. This pattern, though common, is for the most part another puzzle that is seldom talked about. (Some cults believe it to be proof that mankind is born to suffer.)

This pattern of suffering—bliss; suffering—bliss, results from our physiology innocently doing what it has been designed to do. Physiology heals and repairs. Any trauma still with us must be registered in physiology. When the results of trauma (the twist in physiology, the record of the event) are released there must be 'tangible gunk' that must be excreted. (When we sweep the house we raise dust.) And until this impurity is removed from the body we feel 'crappy' (Which is the body's way of sending us the message to clean up the mess.) We may choose to respond with alcohol or other pain killers to deaden the discomfort but what we really need to do, in the first place, is to not encumber the physiology, and in the second place, to assist the body in quickly ridding itself of the debris stirred up by the 'house cleaning'. Proper hydration, breathing, diet, Vedic Exercise and so forth are some of the rudimentary and necessary things we can do but as we are seeing in these later sessions there are some much more powerful approaches to clearing the physiology.

ARE YOU WINNING OR LOSING?

Is "dust from cleaning" being recycled through your physiology only to lodge in another place or are you able to rid your body of the toxicity? Regardless of the efforts you have made since the beginning of the course the understandings of this session may motivate you to make a quantum leap to a more Satvic lifestyle.

There are many adaptations to routine that require minimal time and are enjoyable as well as effective in removing detritus from the physiology. Proper breathing for example is effective in removing toxicity. Vedic Exercise can easily supplant outdated approaches to fitness and help recreate the body. However one very pleasant and powerful technique for both cleaning the physiology and filling the body with joy is to be in the moment.

BEING IN THE MOMENT

While there may be some situation in life that requires our full, undivided attention there certainly must be times available where we are in a relatively safe environment and are able to practice, and become accustom to, being in the moment.[45] Why for example, couldn't we be in the moment while washing an apple? All of life experience, as Eckhart Tolle in his book *The Power of Now* would agree, is an opportunity to step through the portal provided by the Gap into the Now. Following are three games to help you find a way into the Gap and to allow you to become accustomed to being (living) in the gap.

THE GO SLOW GAME

- Choose a time when although you don't have any reason to rush you find yourself rushing.
- For example while you are peeling an apple for the 'apple pie you find yourself rehearsing your acceptance speech for your Nobel Prize and/or Academy Award. Decide to easily get into the present moment.
- Slow down. Breathe deeply through the nose. Slow your movements. Watch the peeler slowly peel the skin from the apple. Move so slowly as to almost stop moving. Watch the paring bend up over the shining blade of the peeler. Watch

as the white (yellow, rose colored) flesh of the apple appears. Notice the wee spots on the skin of the apple—like stars in the night sky. Watch the knife blade, or your hand on the knife handle. Sloooowleeee. Etc, etc, etc.

What happens to your physiology? It slows down. Your breathing slows down. Did you get 'lost in a moment'?

There are some activities where you wouldn't want to practice 'slowing things down': driving a car for example. But there are numerous times when you could play the game. Saying hello to someone. Washing the hands. Polishing shoes. Gardening. Where does the continual need to rush come from? Are we afraid of the Gap? Are we afraid we will feel something we don't want to feel? The benefits of being in the Gap are numerous: physiology slows down; we feel euphoric; we are rejuvenated; the synergy within is given a chance to reestablish itself.

THE SENSORY GAME

Two people can play this game, but it works well with only one.

The instructions and questions are these.

- Close your eyes. What do you hear? For now, just listen—what do you hear? Allow 1 minute. Time it, and when the time is up direct the person to open the eyes and describe what they heard.
- The second person then takes a minute with the eyes closed and listens.
- Then proceed to the other senses—as few or as many as you choose.
- What do you feel? Focus on tactile feelings: what do you feel?

- What do you see?
- What do you taste?
- What do you smell?

Don't let the person beg off with statements like there is nothing to feel. Direct them to feel the clothes they wear—not necessarily with their fingers but feel the shirt collar against the neck, or the shoe pressing against the foot. Give them hints only if necessary.

There is always something to smell, and always a taste in the mouth.

There is no need to rush. The goal is not to smell more smells than someone else. The goal is to get into moment. To get into innocence. To experience and become accustomed to the Gap.

Déjà Vu Game

Do something, and after a brief pause repeat the same activity exactly as before. For example get out of the car and walk into a store. Return to the car and get out of the car again and enter the store. Or have a glass of water— twice. Or get out of bed—return to bed and get out of bed again. Brush the teeth a second time. Are you more alert and alive during the second go round?

These 'games' are a chance to become the silent witness. Don't try to force this. Don't look for it to happen. If it doesn't happen don't beat up on yourself lamenting that something is wrong with you. And when you get into the moment don't try to hold onto it.

SESSION WRAP-UP

Focus for the Week

- During relatively safe activity gently bring your attention back to the moment.

- Practice these games within your group. Have fun, don't make it a chore.

EDITORIAL RANT

I am, as is the culture in general, too serious. Yes a comet could come out of space and do us all in, and I hope someone is figuring out a way to detect and dissolve these dangers. But can I not focus on peeling an apple. Yes there are troubles in Africa. If you are disturbed about the suffering and want to say some prayers by all means do so. If you want to write a check or apply to give service with an NGO this is pretty hard to do while peeling an apple. Wash and dry your hands and go write the check or fill out the application to work in Africa, OR peel the apple. But don't pretend to do both at once—because you will experience neither. Why are we (and I include moi) so reluctant to spend time in the moment? I want to be in the moment.

AGING REVERSAL

- Casting off the residue of 'trauma' can sometimes be uncomfortable.
- Recognize suffering and sickness for what they often are: the release of toxicity.
- The body wants to normalize. It is unlikely to ever quit normalizing. If it does watch out there is a big problem.
- Being in the moment is a very powerful means for promoting aging reversal.

FURTHER READING

Though Eckhart Tolle's book <u>The Power of Now</u> is an excellent understanding of the Gap, and a must read, (You are welcome Eckhart) the issue of the 'how to' of getting into the Gap needs more emphasis. When one is accustomed to being in the Gap the excitement is to tell everybody about the joys of it and to encourage people to get into the 'now'. And for one who is largely living in the gap getting there is delightfully easy. So why would one need games and techniques? Give an easy focus to getting into the Gap.

FURTHER WRITING

Describe a time when you were in the Gap. How did you feel during and after?

***

Session 15: Nature's Gift for Dealing with Trauma has some further good news for dealing with the millstones that may be weighing us down.

Session 15
Nature's Gift for Dealing with Trauma

Vedic thought embraces the idea that the effects of experience on physiology will vary depending on the 'resiliency' of the individual. A harsh experience that may damage one individual may not have much effect on another. Or, for the same individual, an experience that has little effect at one time may have a deeply grating effect at another time. Whatever the case, it would indeed be an unusual person who has lived any length of time without experiencing some degree of trauma.

> ### Erosion
> *It took the sea a thousand years,*
> *A thousand years to trace*
> *The granite features of this cliff,*
> *In crag and scarp and base.*
> *It took the sea an hour one night,*
> *An hour of storm to place*
> *The sculpture of these granite seams*
> *Upon a woman's face.*
> ### E. J. Pratt

Human physiology is fragile. An experience can scar a human nervous system as deeply as a mason's chisel marks stone. The challenge when traumatized is to release the effects of trauma.

What to do? What to do?

For some individuals just thinking about the story of the snake used earlier as example of trauma (*Session 6: Creating Physiology*) may have registered as trauma. In other words noxious byproducts from living may 'wear' away at the physiology. For example a car accident, without resulting in any physical injury, or simply the witnessing of an accident, may result in a 'knot' somewhere in physiology. A horror movie, a loud sound, or some catastrophe viewed on a newscast may do the same. Living can, and usually does, stress and then strain physiology. These experiences result in strain in the same sense as the word strain is used in the expression 'I strained a muscle' or 'I strained my back'.

A good example of a physical encumbrance (strain) is a kidney stone. The body will try to normalize (ie, remove) the accretion through the body's system(s) that deal with kidney stones. These systems do their work consuming energy as they attempt to get rid of the stone. (Though the body may encapsulate the stone energy is still expended.) Any strain must be registered in physiology. (Where else could it be registered?) And as a result the physiology expends energy trying to release the encumbrance.

Please note that the same impulse for the body to rid itself of physical abnormality is also at work with 'emotional' encumbrances. The reaction to the residue of emotional trauma is that it is basically the same anomaly as the kidney stone because in fact they are the same problem: they are physical manifestations that shouldn't be lodged in whatever gap they have found as a home.

All systems of our physiology function to attain balance. When there is a great aggregation of items needing attention and the energy required to deal with the accumulation is greater than the energy available, we begin to feel overwhelmed, energyless and tired. We may use the words 'I am carrying the weight of the world', or 'I have gotten old' to describe the situation. What will the body do when faced with this situation? The body will ask for an unusually large amount of rest.

To summarize: the strain of experience registers in our physiology and the body seeks to normalize it. If the strain resulting from the stress is allowed to accumulate, the body's energy is sapped and aging takes place. In this situation the body seeks less strain and more rest. In most instances, particularly in later life, we retire from activity and rest. Through lack of understanding we refer to this condition as old age.

Now that w e understand the problem let's look at the solution.

GETTING RID OF THE EFFECTS OF TRAUMA

There are cults that believe that we are on earth to suffer—often believing that the more one suffers the more the person is loved by God. Is this the case, or is physiology just innocently doing its job?

Other belief systems conclude that we live in a happenstance universe and being traumatized is bad luck. The solution is to have a drink (or a toke or a snort) and forget about the pain. Recently while listening to a popular folk singer I noticed the theme of his songs was repeatedly 'Woe is me, the world has been rough on me', and then after receiving much applause he continued: 'There is no way out, but drinking helps a lot.'

Do we live in a Universe where there is no way out of suffering? These themes of hopelessness permeate our culture from Beowulf to modern day. We clearly understand that we are burdened. We express our suffering quite well. Agreed we are suffering, but we could choose to also understand that we live in beneficent, loving universe, and Nature has provided the means to deal with the strain of living. To think that there is no way out of suffering is a darkly humorous conception when viewed from an Ayurvedic perspective.

Ayurveda's view is that we are designed to heal. Because of this view Ayurveda searched and was able to find an opportunity within physiology to deal with trauma. The following exercise will hopefully demonstrate that each of us has experienced the dissipation of some trauma over the years.

***

EXERCISE

- Returning to your **I. R. Healthy** notebook and consider an experience that once grated on you but now you can recall without emotional pain.
- Choose an experience that you can talk about without your physiology tightening up at the memory of it.
- Consider the change in the level of discomfort from that of the initial experience and consider how these feelings have lessened over the

years. Choose a relatively innocuous experience: initially the effects were at least as grating as a stick scratching on sand but now the effects are more like a hand passing through air.

- Outline in your notebook your memory of the original event and describe how the effects of recalling the incident diminished over the years.

How does this lessening of the effects of remembering the experience take place? Have we simply found a way to dull the pain? Do we become inured to the travesty? Possibly but Ayurveda's conception of healing, suggests that over the years the healing systems within physiology have loosened the knot of trauma and released the toxicity.

It may not be difficult for some readers to find an instance where emotional healing has taken place but for others it may be extremely difficult to do so. If this is the case for you and you aren't working with a partner this might be a very good time to team up with a partner, or you may want to talk to a health care professional before beginning the exercise. Whatever the case choose something easy. Don't choose something that was, and still is, devastating for you.

In our culture we have the expression "Time cures all things." Of course this expression is nonsense. It may be that *during* time, trauma may dissipate. But time—whatever time may be—has no ability to cure. And surely 'all things' are not cured: often people die full of rage and regret. So let's not take the easy route saying that we don't need to deal with the past; that time will take care of it. On the other hand if you or one of your partners, or someone you know, has healed from emotional damage, then this should be a clear sign that human physiology is capable of healing.

***

HOW TO HEAL

To revive and recover from the usual stresses of the day, among other things, we eat, laugh, enjoy, rest and sleep. In addition we may embrace a helpful world view such as assuming that the 'knocks' we receive are not meant to be taken personally—as opposed to assuming that a leaf falling in our path is a certain sign of an angry god. All that we have studied in *The Aging Reversal Course* is available to assist the body to heal. In addition, sleep and dreaming helps dissipate strain. But what can we do to release the large traumas that have accumulated in our physiology? [46]

SUFFERING: OVER AND OVER

Trauma, unless completely repressed, is often recalled and re-experienced many times throughout the years. In some instances it may almost seem that we are being senselessly tortured yet this is simply physiology going about the business of healing. From an Ayurvedic perspective this remembering of the experience, however discomforting, draws our attention to the pain, employing the power of our attention to clean up unwanted debris. These recurrent memories, sometimes seemingly unbearable, are not the punishment they are often interpreted to be. They are simply the result of the body functioning in the manner that it has evolved to function in…or the manner it has been created to function in. The suffering has little to do with the usual explanation such as paying off our karma, or suffering so we can get to heaven, and so forth—it is simply the result of the body healing.

How healing works is this. Our body, in order to focus our attention on imbalance, will have the mind recall trauma (or recall 'the physiology of trauma' even though we may not recall the specific event). This is the natural functioning of human physiology. How could we be created in a different fashion and still heal and function? What a horrible existence if human physiology didn't have the capacity to heal.

Recall an experience that has largely dissipated over the years. You may have found yourself beset with continued unpleasant memories of this traumatic event but these memories became less and less traumatic. The body wants to be rid of abnormality and will continue to recall the memory of it or particularly the physical sensation of it in order to heal. Frustrating though it may be as we try to enjoy life the body will continue to draw our attention to deep rooted strain regardless of how we attempt to squelch the unpleasantness. The New Age expression "What we resist persists." may have some relevance in this regard.

What to do? What to do?

HOW TO DEAL WITH TRAUMA FROM AN AYURVEDIC PERSPECTIVE

Ayurveda's wisdom for dealing with the discomfort of healing is best simplified in the dictum 'Be the silent witness.' When one of these feelings arises simply take a moment and be the silent witness of it. Often what happens in this silent moment is that the attention is drawn to some area of the physiology. What is important during this time is not that one is **thinking** but that one is **feeling**. Feel the feeling and if the feeling localizes in physiology then attend—easily and briefly—to that area of the physiology. The joy is the release. You may likely feel as though a great weight has been lifted and you will likely feel an influx of energy. Sometimes in the West this is explained as being a Paradigm Shift. If in the past you have avoided experiencing the feeling it will likely return. "What we resist persists."

FREUD, AND HIS BOYS (AND GIRLS)

During this process there is no need to figure out what specifically is going on within the physiology, or to know what particular trauma the discomfort represents. Freud, and Louise Hay, and most of western psychology are far off the mark of usefulness in wanting to understand what a given ripple in physiology signifies. To know doesn't add, and the thinking may take away from the healing process. Ayurveda recommends feeling and witnessing, effortlessly and briefly. To wandering around in the intellect is not conducive to the act of feeling—feeling the body is what is needed. Never mind playing the wise psychologist—how could this be of any use other than an opportunity for stroking the ego?

On the other hand you may know strongly and intuitively, exactly what is being released. If this is the case then fine, but don't distract your attention from feeling whatever it is the body wants you to feel. It may somehow be a thrill to know what the feeling 'means' but what is most important for healing is to put attention easily on what is available to be felt. **It is the process of our attending that does the healing not our intellectual understanding of what is going on.** Our intellect in this instance, as is so often the case, is likely a tool of an ego that is completely terrified of any change and the result is that we do more thinking (what the ego loves to do) and less healing (what the ego doesn't love to do).

A second dictum from Ayurveda is appropriate at this point: 'Take it as it comes.' 'Take it as it comes' means that we don't go rooting around for these feelings. It means that the body will know when the time is right to release a strain. If there is another bundle of strain to be dealt with the body, in it fierce desire to be unencumbered, will present this new package to us—probably all too quickly for our comfort. 'Take it as it comes' means that when we feel sadness, grief, rage, regret or any of the 'negative emotions' we simply feel whatever there is to feel and move on. We don't need to micro-manage the body. On our 'own' volition we don't wallow around in grief or rage. We don't 'call up' more of the same by dwelling on some traumatic experience. If we find that we are becoming overwhelmed we quickly, without delay, seek professional help.

A DIGRESSION

From the above understandings the suspicion may arise that we set up our lives in order to feel what we need to feel in order to get rid of our 'stuff' and move on. It may seem that 'we' (ie, the ego prodded by our physiology) set up our 'Dark nights of the soul'. This is very likely the all too humorous case. The idea that God micro-manages things seems outlandishly farfetched. And that we are the 'playthings of the gods' is another bit of nonsense created 3000 years ago by an ignorant warrior culture. A much more supportable explanation of the human condition is that, if we are in the grip of anything it is that we are puppets to the needs of our physiology. (How to deal with the tyranny of our physiology is discussed below and in **Session 16: The Trouble with the East,** and **Session 18: Quantum Mechanics and Human Physiology**.)

As of now, you have worked with your group and completed the exercise regarding a trauma that has dissipated. You are able to recall the experience without having shockwaves rippling through your body. The key understanding of the exercise is that physiology has the capacity to heal emotional, as well as physical damage.

Try this next exercise.

***

THE AGGRAVATION EXERCISE

This is another relatively safe exercise that will get you in tune with feeling the direction and intelligence of your physiology.

Choose something that you do that you find aggravating.

An example of what aggravates me is to leave work unfinished. To begin weeding a row in a garden and to leave part of the row left unweeded bothers me. In order to feel this feeling I purposely leave a row partly unweeded. I take a break, sit in the shade with a refreshing drink and look at the unfinished row. I keep my attention easily on the unfinished row and feel whatever feelings arise. I don't 'wallow around' in the feelings. I don't go out of my way to question why I feel whatever I am feeling. Nor do I make a judgment that I am stupid to feel uncomfortable about an unfinished row. These and any number of thoughts may occur: 'why am I like this? It must be because my mother, father, brother, uncle, aunt, sister, teacher, coach/ said, looked, stepped on, took/ my ball, hat, pen…etc, etc, etc. What is the use of all this analysis? What I really need to do is to **feel**, lightly and briefly, whatever comes. 'Whatever comes' means whatever my physiology puts on my plate.

(It is odd that over the years I would feel aggravated about an unfinished row, but not concerned in the least that I let myself be thirsty, aching and tired as I feverishly continued to work in the hot sun disregarding the needs of my physiology?)

Set up a situation in order to experience aggravation. Notice over a number of times practicing this exercise if the aggravation lessens in degree.

This is a fun experience to discuss with a partner. The first attempt at it may produce aggravation of the teeth—grinding variety. Later the exercise may seem not so aggravating and later may be only mildly irritating. Later still the exercise may seem ludicrous, and finally riotously humorous.

Repeat the exercise a number of times with at least a day in between sessions. It may take months or years to make some progress. It is in some cases merciful that physiology is built in this fashion.

This exercise is another good opportunity to experience the healing power of our attention.

***

Poof, Gone

Earlier in this session a good night's sleep was sited as a means of releasing the stress of the day. In **Session 12: The Gap** the deep rest of Transcendental Consciousness was cited as Nature's gift for removing deep rooted strain through the deep rest of this fourth state of consciousness. The long drawn out suffering of chipping away piecemeal at blocks of strain may be largely eliminated by finding a way to frequently transcend.

The experience of Transcendental Consciousness as described in Wordsworth's poem is reported in all times and all cultures: Saul on the road to Damascus; a marathon runner finding the 'zone'; the football player mentioned in **Session 10: Vedic Exercise**, a poet becomes enraptured with the symmetry of a berry. While seldom discussed these experiences are commonplace.

A yogi, laughing joyfully, told a story of a man who while sitting in a field eating watermelon, and has an earth shaking transcendent experience immediately jumps up, strides off to the city to inaugurate The Church of the Holy Watermelon.

What happens during these experiences is that we come away feeling cleansed and invigorated. We may feel as though God has touched us. Or that God has filled us with Divine Grace. Or on a milder scale the heart has had a pleasant flutter. Having these experiences regularly in our life is Nature's gift for dealing with the effects of Trauma.

While remembering these experiences of Transcendence our physiology reminds us that we desire more of the unboundedness.

Barter
Life has a loveliness to sell,
All beautiful and splendid things,
Blue waves whitening on a cliff,
Soaring fire that sways and sings,
And children's faces looking up,
Holding wonder like cup.
Life has a loveliness to sell,

Music like a curve of gold,
Scent of pine trees in the rain,
Eyes that love you, arms that hold,
And <u>for your spirit's still delight,</u>
<u>Holy thoughts that star the night.</u>
Spend all you have for loveliness,
Buy it and never count the cost;
For one white singing hour of peace
Count many a year of strife well lost,
And for a breath of ecstasy
Give all you have been, or could be.
Sara Teasdale

Few will agree to 'sell all they have' and there is no need to do so. Nor do we need to witness towering waves spectacularly crashing on a cliff. Walt Whitman rhapsodizes about seeing the universe in a raspberry. Our attention while peeling an apple, or on any other 'mundane task', will allow for the same opportunity of Transcendence.

Entire books have been written about one experience of Transcendence—where for example, breathing slows or stops momentarily prior to sleep. Some individuals found these experiences terrifying; others reported rapture. Understanding what is taking place may increase the chances for an experience of rapture. But it is important to note that for some few individuals Transcendence may be a disturbing experience. I recall a person reporting that having no thoughts was most unsettling—something she never wished to experience again. How unfortunate. Again, it is good to have a group to discuss these issues with, or in this case someone who is properly trained to talk about these experiences.

SESSION WRAP-UP

FOCUS FOR THE WEEK
- Know that Transcendence and the physiology that goes with it are always available for each of us.
- Attend to whatever innocently comes to awareness, effortlessly and easily.

EDITORIAL RANT
Group and cults and sects that understand some portion of the above and employ severe methods for working through trauma are for the most part run by egomaniacs who don't understand the delicacy and fragility of human physiology. The idea that easily putting ones attention on discomfort is a useful thing to do may be all too easily extended to the practice of adding force into the equation: sort of like power yoga. Buyer beware!

AGING REVERSAL
- Releasing the encumbrances of traumatic experience requires deep rest.
- Transcendence provides deep rest.
- Physiology craves Transcendence.
- In this instance give your body what it craves.

FURTHER READING
The poet Rumi. Walt Whitman. Maharishi Mahesh.

FURTHER WRITING
In your **I R Healthy** notebook *describe an instance where you experienced Transcendental Consciousness:* a time when your physiology was slowed to the point of stopping yet you were alert as you have ever been. It may have been a spiritual experience for you. Or it may have seemed very

primal. It may have lasted for only a split second or it may have gone on for days. It may have become permanent. (If so contact me, I'd like to talk.)

***

How to bring Transcendence regularly into our lives is the topic of **Session 16: The Trouble with the East, and the Trouble with the West**.

Session 16
The Trouble with the East and The Trouble with the West

"WATER, WATER EVERYWHERE AND NOT A DROP TO DRINK."

India, generally speaking, is mired in ignorance. They have saints and sages who would readily understand the concepts outlined in *The Aging Reversal Course* but most of the population of India would not.

The West, with its germ warfare mindset, is even more deeply mired in ignorance. There are individuals of a Satvic nature; numbers of them no doubt enlightened, but for the most part we Westerners are alligators walking around disguised in human bodies.

Why make these judgments? Not out of malice but instead to say that most of what India believes and most of what the West believes is dangerous to the well being of the human race. It is not to be disparaging of the people promoting the nonsense—on the contrary, in most cases they are well intentioned and just doing what they need to do. I make these judgments only as a caution.

Most of the 'spiritual' practices that come out of India are from a tradition designed for recluses and are not suitable for 'householders'. The concepts from Ayurveda and **The Aging Reversal Course** regarding sensuality are not suited to a monastery, yet these are essential for people active in the world as they are key to progress and a happy life. How, in fact, could we avoid sensuality and why would we want to—particularly now that we know its purpose is to enliven Life?

From the East there is an understanding of four requirements for the householder: Kama, Arthra, Dharma and Moska. These requirements are seen as essential for a complete life, but seldom, if ever, are they taught to Westerners. On the contrary what are most often promoted are withdrawal, asceticism, vegetarianism, celibacy and austerity, all of which may work well in a monastery but are not useful to most individuals immersed in an active life.

And a notion that seems to pervade all religions and sects is that there is something wrong with activity. The ego's desires must be squelched. That anything undertaken on the basis of the ego is simply done to satisfy some sinful need of the corrupt flesh. This concept that all actions are based on some weakness or fear may be absolutely correct—nonetheless I need to act. I have a purpose in life (Dharma) and on that basis I need to give service to the world family, regardless of how much I am driven by ego. The instruction from most of the 'spiritual' sects of both East and West is the injunction to not trust the 'flesh', and to withdraw from activity. This is an excellent way for a society to fall apart. It also shows little recognition that householders require activity in order that their physiology becomes accustomed to functioning in progressively higher states of consciousness gained through Transcendence. Activity is essential for progress.

In addition, the notion that thoughts (which we blame on the mind) keep us from being in the moment and from being enlightened is often promoted by these traditions. From this understanding the religions and cults conclude that the mind should be silenced. The usual meditation practice resulting from this mindset is one that encourages banishing thoughts. The most destructive of all the component of the monastic way of life (for the householder) are these types of reclusive meditation techniques so often promoted in the West. Both of these approaches (withdrawing from activity and stilling the mind) arise out of Dark Age ignorance. The stress of these reclusive practices increases strain in an already strained life and the result is an aged physiology robbed of vitality.

Few individuals have the capacity to banish thoughts. It is good that we have thoughts as two thoughts are required in order to have the Gap between them. But when we find ourselves in that glorious place of no thoughts we note that the experience is spontaneous and effortless (and upon noting this, the experience is most often over). [47] (Note too, that we have gone to the other extreme in Western culture where we find a television set in most every room, musak in the elevator and other constant sources of noise.)

Further and compounding the problem of reclusive meditations is the use of inappropriate, little understood and mispronounced mantras evoked during the meditation practice. This of course, greatly compounds the misery of improper meditation. Om or Aum for example is a recluse mantra that promotes asceticism and withdrawal. This mantra is possibly suitable for someone living in a cave but hardly suitable for a person with a career and raising a family.

I think most would agree that to have the experience of restful alertness as described by Wordsworth, Dr. Wallace, and numerous others from all ages and places, during a brief morning and evening meditation, would be a wonderful addition to one's daily routine

In the preceding sessions we have presented the benefits of experiencing this consciousness, and posited that meditation particularly, and to some degree prayer are an opportunity to 'settle into' the transcendent. *The Aging Reversal Course* does not fall into the trap of teaching Meditation through a book and yet because of the concerns outlined above I have included below some directions regarding what to avoid and what to seek in a meditation practice.

.

MYTHS ABOUT MEDITATION

MYTH 1) IN ORDER TO LEARN TO MEDITATE AND THEN TO PRACTICE MEDITATION ONE MUST ACCEPT A SET OF BELIEFS.

I have no objection to a person believing whatever it is that they need to believe. But the question arises: why does one need to believe something in order to meditate? Possibly an aspirant likes the beliefs promoted by certain group: say, for example 'God has purple ears'. This belief resonates well and thinking this thought fills the heart with joy. Hail joy! But why would this or any other belief be a requirement in order to meditate?

Human physiology doesn't need to believe something in order to meditate any more than one needs to believe something in order to breathe or eat or swim. We learn and we do.

MYTH 2) MEDITATION IS DIFFICULT

The myth in brief is: Be prepared to struggle—the mind must be controlled—thoughts must be controlled.

Question: If we are struggling are we meditating?

What we have seen in this course is that the body, if we don't mess things up by trying to micromanage, magically takes care of us in an easy and effortless fashion. Meditation too should be easy and effortless. Once one is shown how to allow transcendence to happen then one simply does some little, easy thing and transcendence is allowed to happen.

MYTH 3) TO MEDITATE ONE MUST CONCENTRATE.

Or meditation requires concentration. (This is an extension of Myth 2.)

I heard the Canadian Poet, Earl Birney, speaking years ago about the creative process. He reported an instance that happened while he was mentally searching for a word to give a sense of the emotion he wished to convey in a poem he was writing. He reported that after a time the word he was looking for 'appeared' effortlessly, almost magically. The time Birney had spent in concentration seemed to him to be only a few minutes but it had taken 10 or 15 minutes of clock time. (This is reminiscent of the earlier poem *Asleep on Horseback*.) Notice that though concentration usually means struggle Birney's experience was effortless. Effortlessness is what is needed and how could effortlessness be forced?

Effortless focus is the result of proper meditation technique, not the cause. (And effortless won't happen if we sit around looking for effortless to happen, saying 'Come on. Come to papa! Here effortless. Where are you baby?) To repeat: Effortless focus is the result of proper meditation, not the cause.

In addition, what is the sense of beginning the day, or coming home after a long day at work, only to struggle through a meditation? Is this what our physiology is craving? Indeed, is this good for physiology?

If we have a challenge at work and we need to focus there is nothing wrong with concentration when it is needed. And there is nothing wrong with concentration when it is effortless. But to sit twice a day and struggle in order to quiet the mind is stressful to the physiology. Anyone who is doing this, if they were at all in touch with their physiology, would know immediately that this approach to meditation is incorrect and harmful.

MYTH 4) MEDITATION IS CONTEMPLATION.

Another erroneous idea is that to meditate we choose a thought—say for example peace—and focus on that thought until peace comes to us. If you wish to do this go right ahead, but is this meditating? How can one transcend when one is focused on a leaf on the ocean surface?

MYTH 5) MEDITATION TAKES A LONG TIME

Another myth promoted by the reclusive folks is that meditation should be practiced for numerous hours each and every day, for decades and decades. Would Blake, or Po Chu-I, or Wordsworth or Saint Augustine, agree? They each had a profound experience in a split second—when they were not meditating.

In fact, for householders, meditation is best practiced for a set amount of time: 10, 15, 20 minutes once in the morning and once in the evening. The two sessions should be equal in length: two equal sessions are more suited to the needs of the physiology than one long session. The activity that follows each of these sessions allows the physiology to get used to functioning at the increased level of restful dynamism gained during the meditation. Activity is critically essential to proper meditation practice!

MYTH 6) MEDITATION SHOULD BE FREE OF COST

In traditional India the service of teaching meditation was given freely and the recipient would help support the teacher by making a donation. Modern North America and Europe have a radically different economic system than ancient India. A teacher living in our economy needs a livelihood. If this person is self sufficient and can afford to teach meditation without charge I have no objection. But in our culture we pay for service. When we put new roofing shingles on our house we want the roofer and his/her family to have money in order to have a good life: food, shelter, education, health, leisure, a pension plan etc. In our heart we wish these things for people who work for us. In this culture we don't find it odd to pay for services rendered. It is important for our physiology that we have a loving feeling to give to, and to provide the Meditation Teacher with an appropriate livelihood.

MYTH 7) ALL MEDITATIONS AND ALL MANTRAS ARE CREATED EQUAL.

The looks of the monks who have locked themselves away in a monastery for decades often speak loudly regarding the effects of reclusive meditation practices. Even if you do find a happy individual who looks like he hasn't been living on sour pickles for the last 40 years a cave is probably not the best place for most of us.

MEDITATION SHOULD PRODUCE BENEFITS

Though it is not good practice to look for (or demand) benefits from meditation nonetheless over the weeks, months and years of practice, one might expect progress in activity. Deep rest, transcendence and the release of stress should have some beneficial results. What should be the results of meditation? The poet Thomas Dekker expects golden slumbers.

> ### Golden Slumbers
> Golden slumbers kiss your eyes,
> Smiles awake you when you rise.
> Sleep, pretty wantons, do not cry,
> And I will sing a lullaby.
> Rock them, rock them, lullaby.
> Care is heavy, therefore sleep you;
> You are care, and care must keep you;
> Sleep, pretty wantons, do not cry,
> And I will sing a lullaby:
> Rock them, rock them lullaby.
> **Thomas Dekker**

If, during meditation one looks for, or expects, 'golden slumber' it is exceeding unlikely that one will find 'golden slumber'. Is one meditating if one is expecting something? No, in that case one would be expecting. Without inno-cence, (which one cannot try to achieve, or else one would be 'innocencing' rather than meditating) or if one strains, it is unlikely one will 'settle into' Transcendental Consciousness other than possibly through exhaustion.[48] But meditation (or more accurately its unique state of deep rest and alertness) should produce positive results. The proof should be in the pudding: the evidence should be seen in activity. The benefits should be supported by scientific research. (google meditation, scientific research) One's life should improve: better health, more creativity, satisfying relationships; more productivity. Not a better life in the sense that one thinks of oneself as better than the 'Jones' but better in the sense that one's life is more satisfying today than when one began meditating.

If 'the peace that passes all understanding' is what you sincerely seek then expect a meditation teacher to come to you who can teach you to find access to this peace in an effortless fashion. Seek, and no doubt that teacher will come to you. Effective meditation is easy—when it has been properly taught. See **Reading and Websites**: Bloomfield; and MSI.

PRAYER

Prayer is to thankfulness as meditation is to transcendence. What we are really interested in is thankfulness and transcendence—prayer and meditation are the vehicles that, so to speak, prime the pump. While it may take a prayer to remind one of the feeling of thankfulness it is good not to mistake the prayer for the thankfulness.

Shakespeare's highly ironic scene from the play *Hamlet* where Hamlet, wanting very desperately to kill his Uncle/Stepfather, finds him praying, and decides not to kill him as he believes it will be a sure ticket to heaven for this man who has killed his father. When Hamlet leaves the scene Claudius quits kneeling in prayer, stands and says:

"My words fly up, my thoughts remain below,
Words without thoughts seldom to heaven go."

There is much wisdom in these words my dear Horatioes. Ayurveda would agree completely with the Bard that when words fly up, thoughts remain below. Jesus too chastised some group or other for saying the word too much. He also recommended having the innocence of little children.

Prayer, it is claimed, can move mountains. Dr. Larry Dossey, a noted medical researcher, (See **Reading and Websites**) decided to put this notion to the test. He constructed and put into play an elegant research study in order to determine if the ability of prayer to effect change would withstand the scrutiny of Western Science—and it did. The group of Christians used in the study were overjoyed with Dossey's findings, until he repeated the study with a group of atheists, agnostics, Muslims, Hindus etc and had the same positive result. Later repetitions of the study by other scientists didn't yield the same results as Dossey's studies. Dossey then took to studying the effects of prayer on more easily monitored single celled organisms and was able to demonstrate that some quite natural deterioration in cells could be significantly slowed through prayer.

Ayurveda has long known about the power of thought and early on in **The Aging Reversal Course** the idea that our attention heals was introduced. What is prayer if not attention?

Regarding areas such as forgiveness, or sending love to those we cherish, or feeling love in one's heart for some aspect of the Universe, or feeling love for the entire Universe, prayer may provide great benefits. My intent is not to teach prayer any more than my intent earlier was to teach meditation. But if one has interest towards prayer then it seems, as in any other endeavor that it makes good sense to use one's time effectively.

One very clear insight of Ayurveda is that prayer from a person who is rested and dynamic (as for example Wordsworth's narrator) is likely to create more effective results than if a person's physiology was tired and strained. There are numerous beautiful prayers from all cultures and all times and while the prayer itself may be beautiful and Life supporting a second key component to prayer is that the person saying the prayer has the qualities associated with Transcendence.

FORGIVENESS

In **Session 5: Creating Physiology** the discussion of varying reactions to the snake indicate that the way one chooses to view events creates physiology. As an example of this, Hamlet says that *Denmark is a prison: thinking makes it so.* This isn't to say that forgiveness is wishing an event away by thinking it didn't happen. It is to say we can view the event as trauma that we have the capacity to heal. We don't condone a wrongdoing, but to hold rancor in the heart towards another (regardless of how monstrous the crimes) damages our physiology. We let go of the rancor. We forgive.

In addition, we forgive our self for our transgressions against our self and others. Who has not done something hurtful? Who can cast the first stone? We need to consider that we are not today the person who did whatever it was we did yesterday. Forgive yourself as well as those who have trespassed against you and let the bliss of Life flow through your physiology. And though we may need to say some words in our head, forgiveness takes place in the physiology—in the heart.

SESSION WRAP-UP

Focus for the Week

Find a way to more often bring Transcendence into your life.

Editorial Rant

Caveat Emptor! Beware of 'no pain, no gain' meditation teachers.

Aging Reversal

How effectively can aging be reversed without increasing the experience of Transcendental Consciousness in our physiology? And why pass up the gift of deep peace that the poets and saints describe so well.

Further Reading

Bloomfield.

Further Writing

Describe a time when prayer had a noticeable effect.

***

The quality of the day is set in place the previous day is the theme of *Session 17: From the Mud Comes the Lotus.*

Session 17
From the Mud Comes the Lotus

THE DAY BEGINS THE PREVIOUS DAY

The quality of one's day is largely set in place by the activity of the previous day.

2 A.M to 6 A.M., and particularly the time just prior to dawn, when the earth is lively and nature is on the move, is the best time to awake and arise. Arising at dawn fills the physiology with the qualities of that time of day. This is a time for hygiene, stretching, greeting the dawn, meditation, prayer, followed by a light breakfast, exercise and work.

Noon is the time for the main meal of the day.

Late afternoon Vata time is a time for a brief rest, second meditation and planning the coming day.

Sunset begins Kapha time. A light savory supper prior to sunset if possible, merriment, family time and then off to bed prior to the beginning of Pitta time in order to support the immune system in its endeavors to heal and repair the body.

This routine sets up the physiology for the best possible results in the coming day.

To try to live any other way, on a regular basis, is folly.

To try to begin the day on the morning of the day through the use of stimulants and painkillers is just more of the stupidity promoted by our pop culture and the advertizing industry.

IS IT OKAY TO PARTY?

Of course we can party. All traditional cultures have celebrations, and nights of revelry. Householders are not meant to live like monks: enjoy celebration and festivity, but not night after night, or even weekend after weekend.

FROM THE MUD COMES THE LOTUS

Perfect digestion is to be prized according to Ayurveda. The cautions not to eat anything difficult to digest (brown rice, almond skins or fruit peels) and the caution to not overeat are based partly on the desire for perfect digestion. Poor digestion and the ama [49] that results from it are thought to be at the basis of nearly every disease. Couple this with the concept that Ojas, the essence of Life is the most refined byproduct of perfect digestion. Much like the nutrients in the mud that become the sap that feed the lotus, Ojas feeds the Lotus within human physiology.

The key then, it would seem, is perfect digestion. [50].Every concept and practice of *The Aging Reversal Course* is an aid to perfect digestion. A complete evacuation of the bowel in the predawn Vata time of day would be one indicator of perfect digestion. What then may be added at this stage in the course to further promote digestion?

TRIPHALA

Of all the herbs in the Ayurvedic herbal pantheon triphala is, for most people, the most helpful herb for promoting perfect digestion. But first some general comments regarding the use of herbs.

Herbs are food. Nonetheless most quality products will state on the label: 'Persons with known medical conditions should consult a physician before taking this or any other dietary supplement.' While the chances of herbs adversely interacting with a medication or exacerbating a medical condition may be a rare event nonetheless consult with your doctor if you are on medication or have a medical condition.

In addition, it is not wise to ingest several herbs or herbal preparations unless instructed to do so by a qualified Vaidya. A Vaidya will ask if you are under the treatment of a Medical Doctor, and if you are they will recommend you contact them regarding the addition of dietary supplements. Consulting your doctor still applies if you have a medical condition regardless of what the Vaidya recommends.

As herbs are food they should be consumed in the same manner as food. That is, they should most often be taken with other food, usually at the end of a meal, and most often with water. Your Vaidya will advise.

If a person has poor digestion—that is, they are not digesting food and not assimilating nutrients—it is likely also that herbs will not be digested and the nutrients not assimilated. (This may give new meaning to the expression of 'money down the drain'.) For an alternative approach to ingesting herbs see **Reading and Websites,** Vaidya Mishra's Transdermal System for applying the herbs directly to skin.

To begin a herbal regimen triphala may be the best herb even if you have relatively good digestion but particularly if you have poor digestion. Composed of three berries its effect is neither that of a harsh laxative like senna or a promoter of bulk like psyllium though it does a bit of both. It is a food, high in vitamin C and numerous nutrients and it cleans, detoxifies and strengthens. (See **Reading and Web-sites** Dr. Michael Tierra regarding herbology.)

Will Triphala improve your digestion on the first day of use? It might, but try it for a month. Will it 'fix' digestion of a person following none of what the **The Aging Reversal Course** has recommended? Possibly but…

Also listen to your body. If you don't like the taste of it, don't take it. (Sorry for repeating this again.) I have not heard of anyone not liking Triphala but this may be the case for some individuals.

SESSION WRAP-UP

FOCUS FOR THE WEEK
- Focus on perfect digestion.
- Review your daily routine.

EDITORIAL RANT
Less than perfect digestion will result in impurities (ama) being produced which clogs and putrefies thereby damaging the physiology's intelligence.

When systems and organs of the body lose their intelligence (often the large intestine may be the first instance where this occurs) they begin to function improperly. In the case of the large intestine it 'forgets' how to operate properly and allows substandard materials be used to rebuild the body. The result is aging.

AGING REVERSAL
- Perfect digestion is key to aging reversal.
- The creation of Ojas which is the result of perfect digestion is also paramount to youthfulness and vitality.

- Herbs have memory or intelligence which they 'give' to the physiology.

FURTHER READING

Chopra, <u>Perfect Digestion</u>. Vaidya Mishra's website.

FURTHER WRITING

How about 'The best bowel movement ever'? That will make for an interesting discussion.

***

In **Session 18: Quantum Mechanics and Human Physiology**, we will see that trauma to the 'heart' is at the root of disease and aging. See **Bibliography** Gabor Mate.

Session 18

Quantum Mechanics and Human Physiology

SMALLER THAN THE SMALLEST IS BIGGER THAN THE BIGGEST

To further our discussion of Aging Reversal we now look to the most recent understandings of Physics and particularly Quantum Mechanics.

In 1965 when I was taking the bonehead math course for English Majors the professor was certain that the continued use of particle accelerators to smash minute particles of creation would eventually reveal a primary 'bit' of matter that was the basis of all creation. The key point of his argument was that this bit and the entire Universe were essentially matter.

At the time, as it does today forty something years later, this idea struck me as odd. As progressively finer levels of creation are observed we continue to find seeming 'bits' but upon inspection they are found to be energy and intelligence. Why then would we expect this pattern to suddenly change and matter to turn up? Granted, at first look, the newly found bits often appear to be matter much in the same way our bodies, a tabletop or a rock appear to be matter. But upon closer inspection the bit that so convincingly looks to be matter is found to be vibration. Where is the basis for thinking that these bits of vibration will eventually have matter as their constituent building block?

Quanta, each many tens of millions times smaller than an atom, are vibration. Quantum Mechanics sees everything as vibration manifested from a unified field of oneness. (See **Reading and Websites:** John Hagelin) Vedic thinking has always recognized the conception that everything in the manifest universe is intelligence. Key to the coming discussions is the fact that vibration, when it has a functioning eardrum available becomes sound.

RETURNING TO YOUTHFULNESS

How are these notions of any help in returning a body to a condition of youthfulness? From an Ayurvedic perspective aging occurs when the body forgets, or loses, its intelligence—particularly the intelligence of how to rebuild itself. This intelligence is the instructions encoded as vibrations that direct the rebuilding of every part of physiology. Loss of intelligence happens when the correct (vibration) sound—the information—is forgotten, or distorted, because of toxicity or damage within the physiology. While it is popular to blame 'aging' for aging we may consider that an amoeba has a linage of millions of years (that is billions of reproductions) and amoebas have accurately retained the memory of how to exactly rebuild their progeny. True the amoebas that didn't reproduce accurately died out but an astounding number of amoebas 'parents' accurately retained their memory throughout eons of time.

RESTORING THE BODY'S INTELLIGENCE

Is it possible to restore the body's intelligence? Each of the practices taught throughout the course has been designed by the sages of Ayurveda in order to do just that. Following are additional more powerful approaches that have not been discussed thus far. The body, being self interested in healing and youthfulness, is very much in favor and accepting of these techniques.

NATURE'S ABILITY TO HEAL

Recall a time when you were immersed in nature for a full day. Recall sailing perhaps, or just being out in the wind, water, sunshine and blue skies. Or a day of hiking or mountain climbing may come to mind: dark green spruce trees give way to scree slopes, grey and snow capped mountain peaks contrast startlingly beautiful against a blue sky. The memory of the sight takes the breath away so to speak.

How did you feel during that day and for many days after? Expansive? Dynamic? Settled? Clear? Orderly? Creative? Fully awake? Fully alive? Pure? Bountiful? At peace with the world? (See **Reading and Websites** Pat Morrow, regarding his energizing experience of oneness while climbing.) Why are we likely to experience these qualities after being immersed in nature? And why are these feelings less likely to be available to us during frenetic rush hour traffic?

We have the expression in English, "I felt close to nature." In Quantum Theory there is a notion that the act of observation effects that which is being observed, and during the process of observation the qualities of the observed effect (rub off on) the observer. There is a similar notion in

Vedic thought: that contact with the Unmanifest enlivens the Unmanifest; and a person who contacts the Unmanifest (the Transcendent) is enlivened by the qualities of the Unmanifest.

THE POWER OF THOUGHT

High School chemistry shows that at progressively 'deeper' levels of matter 'things' become more orderly and similar. Gold and lead, other than a few electrons, are nearly identical—startlingly so.

In addition there is progressively more energy at these subtler levels. Burning a lump of coal releases energy: splitting an atom from within the lump of coal releases a far greater amount of energy.

Spending a day immersed in nature usually results in a blissful, euphoric state. If one could contact Nature at a deeper more powerful level than experienced during a walk in a forest the results would be even more profound. Contacting the Unified Field, the subtlest and most powerful level of creation is in fact what happens during Transcendental Consciousness. The qualities of TC—the restful dynamism—are the qualities of the Unified Field. The Unified Field is completely at rest yet completely dynamic. This contact is the most powerful opportunity for aging reversal. The notion from Vedic thought, and now from Western Science, that the observer and the observed take on and enliven the qualities of each other is the basis for the key concept first discussed in **Session 3** that our attention enlivens—our attention heals. Contacting the Unified Field enlivens the Unified Field and also the experience enlivens the individual making that contact.

HUMAN PHYSIOLOGY HAS THE CAPACITY TO EXPERIENCE THE UNIFIED FIELD

If one were to compare a description of the Unified Field and a description of human physiology it becomes clear that they are structured so that human physiology is capable of contacting and experiencing the Unified Field. (See **Reading and Websites** Nader and Hagelin.)

The benefits of meditation—specifically the benefits of Transcendental Meditation as supported by numerous studies and particularly through meta-analysis (www.tm.org)—are similar to the characteristics of the Unified Field. This is to say that the experiencing of the Unified Field during meditation infuse the qualities of the Field into the physiology of the practitioner. It is important to make the distinction that it is the experience of the Field that creates the results: proper meditation facilitates having the experience, but it is not the meditation that is primarily responsible for the results.

A Quote from the Poet Rumi:
'There is a field I will meet you there'.

Consciousness, if you will, is an excellent and indeed essential means of assisting our body to regain its intelligence. And within that Field we are all one and when one of us heals then the earth and all of us heal.

REGAINING INNER INTELLIGENCE THROUGH MANTRAS

The following comments regarding Mantras are surprisingly similar to the comments regarding Herbs.

Though mantras are thought of as words, and more accurately as sounds, they are vibrations. From and Ayurvedic perspective the human body and the entire Universe is the grandest of symphonies imaginable. If we knew the mantras that kept the symphony that is the body in tune we could keep the music playing beautifully tuned to the most delicate note. If we knew the 'sound' of a body part that had been damaged we could help to heal it by properly introducing the accurate vibration. In addition to these 'sounds of the body', there are mantras that draw our attention to the Unified Field: 'Keys to the kingdom of heaven,' if you will. [51]

Given that mantras produce effects (the vibrations of tuning forks influence one another) it is important that mantras are what they purport to be and not mantras to promote a reclusive life, or something else equally as undesirable. Second, it is important that the mantras be 'pronounced' properly, as an incorrect 'pronunciation' would result in a different effect than intended. And thirdly it would be essential in order to be effective that the mantra was 'invoked' [52] in a proper manner. Jesus' dictum regarding 'saying the word too much' comes to mind.

There are numerous types of Mantras and they are often given out willy-nilly (even in books) with little understanding of their purpose, or effects. If we agree that thoughts have power, as we surely must, it becomes very important that **any mantras used should be a correct mantra for the task at hand; correctly 'pronounced'; and correctly 'invoked'.** There are teacher available who have been trained these requirements: There are others who have never considered these concepts. Caveat Emptor!

THE USE OF FOOD AND HERBS TO REGAIN INTELLIGENCE.

Nutritious, Life supporting foods and herbs have maintained the intelligence of how to properly rebuild themselves over the eons, similar in accuracy to the amoebas discussed earlier. When we ingest intelligent food we bring its intelligence into our physiology. (When we ingest dumb and dead and/or genetically altered food we bring its qualities to our physiology). In Ayurvedic thought, at the time of the creation of any part of the body, a corresponding food and/or herb was created that has the corresponding intelligence (vibration) of the body part. Revived Ayurveda [53] offers a huge understanding of the specific herbs suitable for healing the various systems and organs of the body by restoring the body's original intelligence.

It is important to note that treating a symptom rather than the entire physiology is exactly the trap Western Medicine has fallen into. It may be necessary to treat the liver but to do so without treating the entire symphony is unlikely to be successful in the long term. Treat the entire physiology first and then the specifics.

CAUTIONS REGARDING HERBS.

The Ayurvedic understanding of the effects of the vast array of herbs (and combinations of herbs) on human physiology is a vast and complex area of study. The dictum 'A little knowledge is a dangerous thing,' may apply to most of the large array of individuals (among them doctors and pharmacists) willing to recommend herbs. Caution is advised. Even though herbs are food it would be a hard to guarantee that combining herbs with western medications would not create a problem.

- If you are going to take herbs as well as pharmaceuticals consult with your medical practitioner prior to taking the herbs.
- If you are not on meds and wish to begin taking herbs consult with a reputable, well trained, Vaidya.
- If you are going to begin taking herbs on the basis of your own research then check the websites in the **Reading and Websites** as they offer the top quality and the most researched herbs on the market.
- Keep your herbal regimen simple. Don't mix numbers of herbs or herbal preparations. (Note that most herbal Rasayanas are already a complex synergy of many herbs. Note also that the western concept of using an 'active ingredient' in isolation is frowned upon in Ayurveda.)
- Usually herbs are best taken after a meal, though most packaging will have instructions.
- Most herbs are best taken with both water and fat.
- Often a clogged physiology will not assimilate herbs. Numbers of people quit herbal programs considering them useless because their body is unable to ingest the herbs. A herbal program is best begun after a Pancha Karma session when the physiology is well cleaned.

Vaidya Mishra's Transdermal Marma System advocates applying the herbs (which have been formulated within Transdermal Creams) directly onto specific Marmas as instructed by a qualified Vaidya.

SESSION WRAP-UP

Focus for the Week

Consider the idea that everything is not only connected but everything in its essential nature is vibration and All is One.

Consider that these bits of vibration that we think of as matter are a distance from the next bit of vibration (in proportion to their size) in a relationship similar to the distances between the galaxies in relation to their size. Our bodies, which float when in space, are mostly space.

Editorial Rant

Quantum Mechanics and the Vedic understanding of the Unmanifest have a far greater potential to change the condition of our world and our way of living than any previous set of constructs in the history of science.

The horrific state of the world is the result of our collective thinking and the resulting actions stemming from this destructive thinking. While we have tried to change our erroneous collective thinking through education, with some success, contact with the Unified Field will result in spontaneous leap forward in consciousness.

The desperate situation we have created is not the result of the work of the devil, or because God doesn't love us, or that we are in a mad universe with nothing to look forward to but suffering. We cling to these excuses in order to keep us from dealing with the suffering and chaos that we, collectively, have created.

Aging Reversal

- The most effective method of creating aging reversal is to contact and imbibe the qualities of the Unified Field into our physiology.

- Proper use of herbs is also an extremely valuable approach to accurately recreating physiology.

FURTHER READING

- We live in a world and a time when there is a technology of consciousness[54].

FURTHER WRITING

Consider and discuss the impact on human thinking and subsequent human history, of the radical 16th century conception of a sun centered solar system. ***Write it in brief.*** Consider too, the possible impact of Quantum Theory. ***Write it in brief.***

***

Session 19: The Trouble with Enlightened People

Session 19
The Trouble with Enlightened People

THE HIGHEST PURPOSE OF AYURVEDA IS ENLIGHTEN-MENT

It is clear that *The Aging Reversal Course* is not a se-ries of tricks that allow a person to live like a hog and peri-odically clean up the mess. Instead Ayurveda encourages us to lead a Satvic life which gradually refines the physiol-ogy so that in a flash of bliss we flip the switch (or allow the switch to flip) and we recognize who we really are—who we have always been. We allow enlightenment.

Upon nearing enlightenment an individual may be-come sick. One saint reported 11 years of sickness prior to enlightenment. Why would these great souls (we are all great souls) become sick? The answer is found in *Session 14: A Millstone* regarding the release of accumulated toxins.

The body releases toxins (sometimes exceedingly noxious toxins) in its desire for balance. The toxins must be eliminated or they may become a home for disease or in some other way debilitate the physiology. This is a well known concept in Ayurveda and according to some Vaidyas and yogis the primary purpose of Ayurveda is to prepare the body to accept and maintain Enlightenment.

If you listen to what enlightened people say about becoming enlightened they seldom speak of disease or suffering. Often they report a dark night of the soul: they had a rough night, woke up, shuffled to the park and there it was—enlightenment. (See **Reading and Websites** Eckhart Tolle, *The Power of Now*.) Or they had spent 60 years in a cave doing 'austerities', and upon hearing a bird sing—kabaam, enlightenment.

It may seem to them that in whatever way they were enlightened is <u>The Way</u> to get enlightened. And if the enlightened are savvy enough to not preach this idea then their disciples often do. By way of example: one great yogi drank lime juice and soon all the disciples were drinking lime juice—whether they had to choke it down or not.

While enlightenment could happen in any fashion it is of course not limited to or brought on by any particular set of circumstances. If it was brought on my some particular set of circumstances someone would remember and we would all be doing exactly what that person did, and quickly become enlightened.

One enlightened person reported that even a very crude person—malicious, and an eater of all kinds of noxious foods—could, if even one of their 'internal systems' was 'refined' enough, become enlightened. I like the idea: anyone could become enlightened at anytime. Who am I to judge otherwise?

THE CELLO

The trouble with enlightened people—from my limited and not so humble perspective—is that they don't know how to play the cello. No doubt they could learn to play the cello, and would probably learn quickly and play beautifully if that is what Nature called them to do. But upon becoming enlightened they don't spontaneously become proficient at playing the cello. And if we were to ask them how one should go about learning to play the cello they probably wouldn't able to tell us very much—other than that one should be in the moment when playing.

Where is this discussion going? My question is: 'Do the enlightened understand Ayurveda any better than they understand the cello?' In most cases they probably don't. What they spend most of their time talking about is what it is like to be enlightened. Usually they will say that becoming enlightened is such a simple and easy thing. So easy—and then they laugh, or smile at the very least, at the simplicity of it all and say: 'It is so easy; all one has to do is to flip the switch—or indeed to let the switch flip. Nature wants us to be enlightened. In fact we are enlightened— we just need to remember.' Tee hee, etc.

I have nothing against any of this. It is all very beautiful. This idea that any one of us could 'slip into' cosmic consciousness now—right now—is a very wonderful, expansive thought. So I have no quibble in reading these people's books or going to listen to them at Sat Sangs in the hopes of becoming enlightened. But what they may not focus on enough is the refinement of physiology.

So with all the above said, do these enlightened people understand Ayurveda any better than they understand the cello? Do they understand that at the time they were enlightened their physiology was probably in pretty incredible shape? They know and will say if asked, that the brutish person discussed earlier who could nonetheless still reach enlightenment, will be much better able to 'slip into enlightenment' were his/her physiology 'clear'. And too, if the physiology is 'clear' the person will have a much better chance of being able to stand the 'voltage' of enlightenment, and remain enlightened.

But on the other hand, I don't want to leave this discussion, as so many proponents of Ayurveda and the Satvic life often do, by saying that what is required to be enlightened is years of grinding austerities to attain purity. Enlightenment is possible for anyone in any condition, at any time and any place but it is usually more likely to happen when one's physiology is reasonably well cleaned up.

Another notion that I don't wish to imply is that we would have been better off to have born to a reclusive life—where we could live a pure life. That we are householders is not an act of blind fate but instead the result of a beneficent Universe. We can lead a pure life and each of us has as a householder our best opportunity to move rapidly towards enlightenment.

My point regarding all the above discussion is: if you are going to listen to the enlightened speak please bring proper hydration and a lunch that will satisfy all the 6 tastes as per the requirements of your physiology on that day.

And with utmost sincerity I express my best wishes to all the Enlightened Enlighteners, and to those of us not enlightened, myself included, best wishes for a speedy Enlightenment.

AGING REVERSAL WITHOUT TRANSCENDENCE

Can aging reversal occur without prayer and meditation—more specifically without the 'silence' that comes from prayer and meditation? I believe the answer is yes, but is aging reversal likely to happen quickly and for as large a number of people without a component of Consciousness in the mix? Possibly yes, but likely no.

THE LADY WHO PRACTICED ZEN BUDDHISM.

Gathered around a table at lunch the discussion came around to revealing our ages. The woman sitting next to me looked young—ageless really. Her skin was pink, her eyes were shining and she moved with grace and youthfulness. Her husband announced that he was eighty three—I wondered if she was sixty. She was seventy six. Later when I had a moment I congratulated her on her youthfulness. She replied that she had been very fortunate that her son had introduced her to Zen Buddhism twenty five years previously. She reported that she arose before dawn every morning and practiced everything that has been recommended in this course.

Am I promoting Zen Buddhism, or this or that meditation, or this or that church, or this or that type of prayer? No, I am promoting 'Silence' and more specifically Transcendental Consciousness however you may choose to reach it. Our time on earth is precious. Find **Silence** and not something that is possibly, you know might be, could be, maybe, Silence.

And in addition to meditation and prayer we can partake of silent surroundings; of being mindful; of listening to our bodies. Learn how to take your pulse through an Ayurvedic practitioner and experience the silence of taking the pulse.

Or include brief periods of silence in your day. For example have no conversation, or radio etc until after breakfast. This doesn't have to be practiced every day but maybe one day a week of silence or one day a week where silence is practiced for an hour. Or one day a month could be reserved for silence. In most traditions there are times for silence.

SESSION WRAP-UP

Focus for the Week

Focus on the silence between all things. Is there 'something' that is truly YOU? Something that observes all else including the mind?

Editorial Rant

It is so wonderful for the family of man to have increasing numbers of enlightened individuals on the earth. There needs to be a book written about them. For example to explain that these individuals could be as dumb as a stone—given that a prodigious intellect has nothing to do with enlightenment and in fact may interfere with allowing it to happen. The business in life of the enlightened may be far removed from being enlighteners—witness the poet Walt Whitman, or the character Larry in the novel The Razor's Edge both these individuals made a living doing odd jobs and had no great interest in enlightening others. (Both these men might or might not have been enlightened, who can say?). And then there are the pretenders to deal with. As if life isn't interesting enough.

Aging Reversal

Aging reversal probably is much easier to accomplish after one is enlightened, but why wait—for either.

Further Reading

Lorne and Lucia Hof, see **readings and websites**.

FURTHER WRITING

Describe an experience where you were 'the silent witness'.

***

A New Age of Life and Light is discussed in **Session 20.**

Session 20
A New Age for the World Family

A CHANGE IN TIME: MORE ACCURATELY A CHANGE IN WORLD CONSCIOUSNESS

In the Greek Drama <u>Philoctetes</u> written by Sophocles over two millennia ago, the main character expresses a belief that is alive and well in our culture today. Philoctetes describes Odysseus as follows: "His tongue will dabble in any lie, he cannot feel remorse, and when he acts, the end is always evil." Later expressing rage against one of Odysseus's comrades the same speaker continues; "The evil in this world never dies.…external powers lovingly protect it. They snatch all that is foul and corrupt out of danger—I think it's a game for them—then down, down, into the grave goes anything fine and good."

The history of the last 3000 years offers many examples to support these sentiments but is this the inevitable way of life? To argue the contrary, that life on earth is going to change—that 'good' will be rewarded and 'evil doers' will lack support—in most circles would encourage ridicule.

My novel ***Before the Dawn*** makes the argument that world consciousness is changing, and dramatically so. Sybil Kalla, a main character in the novel, arrives in the Kings

Court ostensibly to heal him, but besotted with wine she makes this pronouncement:

> She stood, her shoulders thrown back in a dramatic
> pose, and uttered a single word: "Time." And then in
> a devout, hushed voice she repeated the word. "Time.
> Time has allowed us only slaughter and want these
> last thousands of years. Now the Great Mother offers
> a chance…a great opportunity—for Life." (She con-
> tinues speaking after a number of lines of description)
> "today, and for ages into the future, for as many cen-
> turies—more, yes, many, many years more than these
> few thousand years humankind has lived in hell. Now,
> today, we have a great opportunity. Mother Time once
> again protects the good among us."

Later in the novel the King's son meets the first visi-
tors to the Kingdom in 200 years. They have the same
prophesy:

> "Our Mothers tell us that two hundred years have
> passed since the end of the Everlasting War. Now hu-
> mankind will again increase and prosper. Our people,
> and no doubt yours, expect that the way we now live
> is the way life will be. Why would there be a change?
> Only a fool would expect any change. But there was a
> great change two hundred years ago—for your peo-
> ple as well as ours. Two hundred years ago, in a time of
> horror, peace of a sort engulfed our separate lands."

Later in the novel Kalla's sister, the Sybil Pura, expands
on this concept when one of the Windriders asks:

"The 'Character of Time' means what, I wonder?"
Pura responds: "That in this coming age there will be more Life, more strength available for mankind."
"Available to the evil among us as well as the good?" Leason questioned.
"Though not a philosopher, Leason, you ask an insightful question," Pura laughed. "And too, I would talk with you about this idea of evil another time. But yes, the rain waters all plants. Though the misuse of this energy, or if you will allow me, the misuse of the grace of the Divine Mother, will harm the user—much the reverse of the Dark Ages when misuse most often seemed to be rewarded."

(The novel may be found at www.paulcolver.info)

Is there any substantive reason to believe that the world is dramatically changing?

WHAT CURRENT DAY SAINTS AND SAGES HAVE TO SAY ABOUT TIME.

Lorne and Lucia Hof, Eckhart Tolle, Richard Sylvester (*I Hope You Die Soon*) and a holy host of others report that world consciousness is 'waking up'. That is to say, individuals are waking up to their true Self. At the same time they are awakening, and enlivening, our earth with the energy of Life. How is this possible? ***Session 18: Quantum Mechanics and Human Physiology*** presents the principle that the observer enlivens the observed, and as well, the observed enlivens the observer. One of the primary principles of Ayurveda first seen in ***Session 3*** is that our attention heals; our attention enlivens. World Consciousness has been enlivened over the past decades. The world today in early 2010 is changing—dramatically. True, we are walking a precariously narrow tightrope, hovering above another

Dark Age with war and suffering everywhere, but the world is waking up. Will we make it? We will indeed have an answer soon.

FURTHER ENCOURAGING NEWS

One Vaidya from a 5000 year old Brahmin family reported that there are more people meditating in North America than in India.

There are groups practicing advanced meditation techniques in every major city in North America and Europe. There is a group exceeding 2000 of such individuals in the center of the United States.

In the center of India a city, currently partly occupied, is being constructed to house 10,000 experts in enlivening consciousness. Planning is underway to bring this number to 100,000 of these experts in consciousness.

This enlivening of consciousness is the first good news I wanted to report in this final session. You may be part of this consciousness enlivening. If so, my warm congratulations to you. The second great vision is as follows.

THE BEST OF THE WEST AND THE BEST OF THE EAST COMBINED.

Wouldn't it be wonderful to have a Health Care system based on an understanding of valid, reliable knowledge of both the East and the West? Most of the great scientific discoveries have had an intuitive basis. Typically after the initial flash of intuitive insight, rigorous testing is the order of the day to determine the validity and reliability [55] of the notion. Ayurveda is easily able to supply a complete understanding of human physiology—and disease—on an intuitive basis. What a relief it will be to have a system of

Health Care cleansed of the superstition and nonsense—of both East and West—and to be rid of the practice of treating symptoms.

THE TIPPING POINT

Humanity has seen radical changes during the last millennia. In the Dark Ages thugs ruled barbarous fiefdoms throughout Europe. Over the centuries China warred, and Africans enslaved and slaughtered each other. In fact most of the history we know has been a history of a Dark Age. At the time of this writing much of the world lives in horrific conditions—North America and Europe included. But there have been great changes. Labor laws for example, without which the deplorable conditions of the Industrial Revolution would be more widespread than they are today. Seemingly driving these changes are numbers of individual, often in concert but often on their own accord, doing what needs to be done to bring about the change. Anti-slavery laws were put in place with good effect. Americans on the frontiers hung up their six shooters and submitted to the rule of law—an amazing accomplishment when one considers present day Afghanistan or Mogadishu.

In all the instances of great change humanity demanded the change but from my not so humble point of view, Consciousness supported the change.[56] We are at another of the tipping points in world history. Consciousness is ready and humanity is crying out and working diligently for change. Collectively humanity wants the destruction of the planet to cease. Collectively humanity feels that somehow the planet and all on it are one.

I was an ardent member of the movement to save the environment in the 60s, and by the 70s I was sure that we had missed our opportunity that the earth would be destroyed. Today, though the environment is in much worse condition than 40 years ago there is a grand chance to turn earth back into the garden it once was. Today there is a broader understanding that Earth is home—that we all live downstream. Across the planet individuals are focused on loving and repairing our planet. Today there is great energy and consciousness for change.

THE STARFISH

And if all of the above is nonsense then we still have the comfort of the *Story of the Starfish:*

> *One morning after a huge storm a young couple was walking along a beach aghast at the wreckage. They came upon an elderly woman who was picking up starfish one by one and tossing them back into the ocean. The small, frail person appeared ludicrous in her endeavor to clean up the beach and the couple began to laugh in their nervousness. One said, "You can't be serious. You'll never clean up this mess."*
> *The elderly woman bent down, picked up a starfish and pitched it gently into the water and said, "Maybe not, but I sure helped that one." The young couple began gently tossing starfish into the water.*

Whatever happens—mankind returns to the Dark Ages or we enter a glorious age of spiritual and material abundance—someone gently pointed me towards the water. And **The Aging Reversal Course** hopefully is an opportunity for many individuals to begin moving, or to continue moving with greater ease, towards the water. That is my hope.

SESSION WRAP-UP

Focus for the Week and the Days and Years Ahead

- Listen to and trust your physiology.
- Observe and support the numerous Life supporting initiatives underway everywhere on our planet.

Editorial Rant

Our attention enlivens what which we focus upon. In this new age the energy of Life supports those of us of with Life supporting intent.

Aging Reversal

I wonder how effective a person who is not healing themselves can be at healing the planet. The two endeavors are intimately linked.

Further Reading

Pass the course on to a friend. Start a new group and work through the course again in somewhat of a leadership capacity.

Further Writing

Write and thereby have your attention on an instance of the earth being repaired.

Best wishes,

Paul Colver

***

Following are *Appendices A: (Abhyanga), C: (Cooking),E: (Exercise), M: (Marmas), P: (Pranayama), Q: (Questionnaire)*, and the *Reading and Websites* pages.

Appendix A
Abhyanga

ABHYANGA: A PLEASANT WARM OIL MASSAGE FOR SUPPORTING THE IMMUNE SYSTEM.

Following are instructions for Abhyanga: a warm oil massage that is one of the best things you can do to strengthen your immune system and create balance in your physiology.

Light, organic sesame oil is the premier oil recommended by Ayurveda for massage. Of all the oils it is best at opening and cleaning the pores. Sesame oil has a mildly heating effect and may not be suitable to some body types particularly in the summer. Coconut oil may be a better choice for individuals who are constantly hot.

A variety of oils are suitable for massage: almond oil, grape seed oil, olive oil (particularly soothing to sunburned skin).

High quality, organic oil is recommended as pesticides and the like are often fat soluble.

CURING THE OIL

- Pour the oil into a high quality stainless steel saucepan from which you can later easily repour the oil into a suitable container.
- Heat the oil on a medium heat.
- Test the oil by flicking just a few drops of water from the finger tips into the oil. Careful. Do this

periodically as the oil warms until a crackling noise is heard.

- Remove the oil from the heat and allow it to cool enough to pour.
- Be cautious working with hot oil. Do not over-heat. This is probably not a time to practice being in the moment.

PROCEDURE FOR THE MASSAGE

- Set a cup or bottle containing a small amount of oil in hot water and warm the oil to body temperature (or a bit higher or lower to suit your pleasure).
- Perform the massage in a warm place.
- You may elect to cover the floor with a sheet as it is usual to drip some oil during the massage.
- Sip warm water or herbalized tea, and breathe deeply and often during the massage.
- Begin by applying oil to the head. Massage gently with the palms of the hands.
- Be gentle with the face and most gentle with the neck area between the chin and the collarbones. (Your body will know 'instinctively' to avoid rigorous massaging of this area.)
- The feet, legs, buttocks, hands, arms and shoulders can be fairly vigorously massaged if you wish.
- Stomach and chest should be handled fairly gently.
- The back may be vigorously massaged.
- Use circular motions where it seems applicable, particularly over the joints.

- Clockwise motions are highly recommended. That is to say: if someone were looking at you, your hand would be rotating in a clockwise motion from that view. When massaging the back of the body, consider the view as if looking from behind and perform clockwise rotations for this view.
- Use long strokes over the calves, thighs, fore-arms and arms.

Leave the oil on for as long as is comfortable. Shower with warm water and a high quality liquid soap.

The pores of the skin absorb oil and are cleansed by the oil. You will find the skin smoother and you will have a pleasant glow. The aroma of sesame oil is pleasant for most people. If it is not pleasant for you then use alternate oil.

Abhyanga is particularly effective for soothing and balancing Vata dosha.

Enjoy the warm oil massage. Don't rush. If your time is constrained then do less of massage, but in a leisurely manner.

Appendix C
Cooking

There are books available based on Ayurveda that offer up extensive lists of what to eat depending on your constitution; what not to eat at various times of the year; what to eat if you are fat or thin, or old or young, etc, etc, etc. Nothing wrong about this approach but **The Aging Reversal Course** *has encouraged you to focus on listening to what your body wants—and then finding a Life supporting manner to meet those needs.* Eat only food that is pleasing to you.

CHAI

- While 1 ½ cups of previously boiled water is coming to a boil add whole cloves, cardamom pods and cinnamon bark.
- Other spices may be added such as fennel seeds, fenugreek seeds (bitter), ginger root, licorice root, black pepper, mint and/or saffron (add saffron at the last minute).
- Bring to a boil.
- Add 1 tea bag per 1 ½ cups of water. (Use any type of tea you wish: white, green, decaf. (Is decaf tea natural? Oh these weighty questions.)) Keep the mixture at a low boil.
- When the water has been boiling for a while, or has just begun to gently boil, add 1 ½ cups of milk and bring the mixture for an instant to a

gentle boil, and then turn off the heat and let the chai steep. (Boiling the tea is thought to increase the amount of caffine and you may choose to add the tea after the milk has boiled and the chai is steeping.)

- Strain, serve and enjoy.
- Paul's Special Chai: Cloves, cardamom, cinnamon, ginger—skip the tea bag and add instead toasted fennel, coriander and cumin seeds. A dash of mint on a hot day is a nice touch. (This chai suits me: it may not suit you.)

GHEE

Ghee is unsalted butter that has been gently heated to remove the impurities. There is research available indicating the benefits of ghee though I have never taken the time to look it up and read it.

- In a skillet that is easy to pour from, gently heat at a below medium temp a pound or two of unsalted butter, preferably organic.
- When the goop at the bottom of the pan quits bubbling up to the surface—at the same time the 'crackling' will stop—turn the temp to low and let the ghee sit for 40 minutes. A dark golden color is preferred. Ghee that has cooked until it is brown may be okay. Ghee that has been overcooked and looks like motor oil will make good barbeque starter. Careful.
- Strain and retain the 'crust' that has collected on the surface. Discard the scrapings on the bottom of the pan. They also are good firestarter.

Ghee lasts a long time without refrigeration, though you may wish to store it in the fridge. The taste and texture may take some getting used to though I now prefer it to butter. (Particularly when I see what is scraped out of the bottom of the pan.)

LASSI

Lassi is yogurt mixed with water in any portions that suit your taste. Sweeten if you like. Add in toasted cumin powder and salt, or saffron, or any other number of spices. Also sweet fruit may be blended into the lassi.

PANEER

Using a double boiler or a pot within another pot partly filled with water, on a medium heat, not much above boiling temperature and bring whole milk to a light boil. Careful it burns easily—if necessary remove the pot from the heat. Add yogurt or lime juice (or both) and the milk will curdle. If the milk does not curdle the temperature may be too low. If this is the case heat the milk to a little higher temp, stir it, add more lime juice or yogurt and wait for the milk to separate.

When it has curdled and has cooled a bit, strain the mixture through a strainer or cheesecloth. Let the curds drain. Press the liquid (the whey) out of the curds and when the curds are suitably dry set them in a bowl to firm up. Or pat into a cake and when they become firm cut into cubes. The paneer and the whey maybe stored in the fridge for a few days.

Typically paneer, which is high in fat, is eaten lightly fried, mixed with vegetables, at lunch. Sag Paneer which can be a taste treat is cubes of paneer simmered in pureed spinach with spices, particularly turmeric. Seldom is Paneer eaten at supper as it is considered heavy. Whey is considered clogging to the channels but some physiologies may find it acceptable. I find the taste delightful.

Appendix E

Exercise

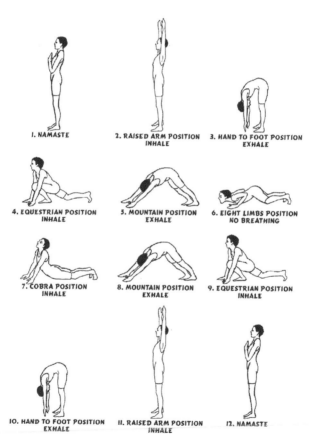

1. NAMASTE

2. RAISED ARM POSITION
INHALE

3. HAND TO FOOT POSITION
EXHALE

4. EQUESTRIAN POSITION
INHALE

5. MOUNTAIN POSITION
EXHALE

6. EIGHT LIMBS POSITION
NO BREATHING

7. COBRA POSITION
INHALE

8. MOUNTAIN POSITION
EXHALE

9. EQUESTRIAN POSITION
INHALE

10. HAND TO FOOT POSITION
EXHALE

11. RAISED ARM POSITION
INHALE

12. NAMASTE

Note that the positions have been drawn to convey what might be comfortable for a beginner. Don't strain. Proper postures include for example an arch to the back in position 1, head closer to knees in #2, the knee joint at 90 degrees but the foot flat on the floor in #4, butt higher in #5 creating more of a peak; hands, chest, knees and two sets of toes equal the eight points—with the rump not so high. This pose is not held for more than an instant.

- *First* posture of the Sun Salutation is to stand (preferably at dawn, facing east) with feet together. (Feet together only for this posture.)
- Hold the hands together in Namaste position (as though in prayer). (Hands together only for this posture.)
- Breathe in and out normally.
- *Second* posture: Allow the hands and arms to fall slowly to the sides, and then raise the arms and hands over the head. Don't strain. Arch the back, but only if it is easy to do so.
- What is going on with your breathing as you do this? (As you raised your arms the rib cage expands: this is a good time to breathe in.)
- *Third* posture: touch the toes. (Easily, do not strain, bend only as far as comfortable.)
- What is going on with the breathing as you do this? (As you begin to bend the rib cage begins to contract and the air is forced out of the lungs. As you continue to bend this is the time to breathe out. By the time you touch the toes (or get as close to them as you are easily able) the lungs should be empty. (Do not lock the knees:

keep them slightly bent forward as you perform this phase of the exercise.)

- Move fluidly into the next posture (extend the right leg (some commentators suggest extending the left first)) and then the next posture, and then briefly 'touch down' in the 8 limbs' position. Then again the cobra, the mountain, the equestrian (again the right leg extended: the left is extended in the second half of this first set), and then smoothly hands to feet.
- Return to the standing position, hands over the head in the second *position*. As you do this the rib cage expands and you breathe in.
- Perform Namaste, breathe normally and then repeat the 12 steps this time extending the left leg rather than the right.
- You will have completed one set. Continue on with more sets as is comfortable, but at the end of the set(s) lay down take a brief rest and allow the attention to focus within the body as it will.

If everything feels smooth and fluid then good. Regardless it is worthwhile to learn this very valuable exercise from a competent instructor.

Appendix M
Marmas

ARE MARMAS CHAKRAS?

Inevitably questions regarding the Charkas arise. How can one enliven the Chakras?

Marmas and Charkas, though sometimes located seemingly together are two different things. My advice is to leave the Chakras alone. All of what you have learned in this course will clean and purify the body, ultimately improving the functioning of the Chakras. The practices you have learned in the course are enough to purify your physiology. If some feeling arises, feel it normally as you feel anything else but don't fool around with the Chakras unless they knock loudly on your door. If you hear a loud knock then get some experienced and trustworthy guidance. For more on Chakras read Margo Ananda and/or visit Langenkamp website.

Appendix P
Pranayama

Pranayama, as with Surya Namaskara and yoga postures, should be learned from a qualified instructor who is not of the power yoga/no pain—no gain school of yoga.

One sits comfortably in a quiet setting unoccupied by any other activity. Using the right hand, the thumb is used to close off the right nostril and the two middle fingers are used to close off the left nostril.

Close off the right nostril, breathe out and then in through the left.

Close off the left and breathe out and then in through the right.

Practice Pranayama for up to five minutes prior to meditation or silent time.

Practice without effort but this does not mean one could not breathe deeply; nor does this mean one should breathe deeply.

Allow some time before going back into activity.

COOLING BREATH

While breathing diaphragmatically through the mouth hold the tongue in a 'U' shape to act as a funnel. Note how the air is cooled as it is drawn over the tongue.

Appendix Q
Questionnaire

Answer the questionnaire on the answer sheet provided.

Relax and enjoy. There aren't correct or incorrect answers.

Don't agonize over answers: complete the first questionnaire relatively quickly.

Record your answers on the **left** columns of the accompanying answer sheet. Include an answer for **each** item A, B, and C of **each** question.

Use of a 9 to indicate a definite 'yes' to the statement. A zero to indicate a definite 'no'.

Use 6, 7 or 8 to indicate lesser agreement than 9.

Use 1, 2 or 3 to indicate greater agreement than 0.

Do not use 4 or 5 as an answer

1)   A—I learn quickly and forget quickly.

B—I learn moderately fast and retain information fairly well.

C—I learn slowly but retain what I learn seemingly forever.

2)   A—I enjoy warm, slightly humid weather.

B—I enjoy cool, brisk weather.

C—I enjoy hot, dry weather.

3) A—My appetite is variable: I eat whenever I can get around to it.

B—My body is like a clock: when it is mealtime I must eat.

C—Once I get started I can slowly eat a huge amount of food.

4) A—My build is slim, (possibly with protruding bones).

B—My build is medium with some muscle.

C—My frame is large and my build is thick.

5) A—My skin is dry and possibly rough

B—My skin is freckled and/or burns easily in the sun.

C—My skin may be: oily, cool, without blemish, very white or pale for my skin color.

6) A—Most of my fingernails may be best described as having an oval shape.

B—Most of my fingernails have an angular shape. Narrower at the base (near the knuckle) and wider near the tip. The nails may be pinkish and flexible.

C—Most of my fingernails have what is best described as a square shape. They may be thick and not easily bent.

7) A—I am able to lie on the beach all day.

B—I must be cautious of the heat.

C—I find cold and damp weather unpleasant.

8) In terms of getting things accomplished I

A—tend to have numbers of things on the go.

B—get things done on time.

C—am relaxed and enjoy the work.

9) A—I like sour and salty food

B—I like sweet tastes (bread, milk, sweets and meat as examples)

C—I like peppery foods (chilies, pepper, and possibly honey)

10) Rate the following senses as above in terms of level of enjoyment (9 signifying that you very much enjoy that sense, etc.)

A—Sound

B—Sight

C—Taste

11) A—I like being in the wind. For example hang gliding, flying a kite, climbing, or sailing.

B—I like cool sports. For example skiing, skating, tobogganing, golfing.

C—I like to be in water. For example swimming, snorkeling, scuba diving.

12) A—My mind is restless and may bounce from one thing to another.

B—My mind is sharp and clear. I know what I need to do and I get it done.

C—My mind is steadfast, at peace, and usually not in a rush.

13) A—My body weight is low

B—My body weight medium

C—My body weight heavy

14) A—My eyes are small, narrow and move quickly and/or blink often.

B—My eyes are penetrating and capable of sharp looks.

C—My eyes are large. The whites may be very white. I may seldom blink.

15) A—I should drink more water.

B—My thirst is often great.

C—I can go for a long time without water.

16) A—Physical activity for me is a must.

B—I enjoy physical activity but less so in the heat.

C—I am slow to get started.

17) A—Worry or anxiety is often possible in my life.

B—Anger, irritability figure in my life.

C—Attachment, or even greed and envy are sometimes in my life.

18) A—Spiritual for me has to do with joy, bliss and zest for life.

B—Spiritual for me is being compassionate and understanding.

C—Spiritual for me is being faithful and/or devotional.

19) A—My beliefs are changeable. I will usually consider new ideas.

B—I believe what the facts support.

C—I hold to my beliefs and I am as steady as a rock.

20) A—My dreams are of flying, jumping, running.

B—My dreams are of anger violence, war.

C—My dreams are of water, swimming, romance

21) A—My sleep is interrupted and light.

B—My sleep is brief but adequate.

C—My sleep is deep and prolonged.

22) A—I spend money quickly.

B—I spend on luxuries, sometimes when I probably shouldn't.

C—I am a saver though I may spend freely on food.

23) A—My pulse is feeble, and/or quick.

B—My pulse is moderate with a bit of a bounce to it.

C—My pulse is slow—like a swan slowly gliding on water.

24) A—My digestion is weak.

B—My digestion is strong and fast.

C—My digestion is slow.

25) A—My hair is fine and dry.

B—My hair may be reddish, blond, thinning or balding.

C—My hair is thick, or coarse and possibly oily.

26) A—I hardly sweat at all.

B—I sweat readily.

C—My skin is often oily.

27) A—I walk in a quick, lively fashion.

B—My manner of walking is brisk and I appear purposeful.

C—I generally walk slowly and enjoy my surroundings.

On your answer sheet add up the totals for each column. High totals in the A column indicate **Vata constitution or imbalance**. B column, **Pitta constitution or imbalance**. And the C column **Kapha constitution or imbalance**.

Compare the totals. One column's total may be larger than the other two totals combined. Or you may have two columns with high totals and one with a much lower total. Or possibly your three totals are approximately equal. All of this will be discussed. If you have totals that indicate a constitution that seems accurate for you then return and complete Session 6.

If you feel the need to spend a few more minutes on your questionnaire then complete the **right** hand half of the answer sheet as per the directions in brackets on the answer sheet. (See "Award a 4 to one space only.") From the questionnaire select the most applicable statement from each of the questions numbers 1 to 27 and place a 4 under one of the columns A, B or C to indicate which statement most accurately describes you. (This is to be answered on the right side of the answer sheet.)

There may be an instance where you feel that 4 should be divided and entered as 2 in two columns. Or in some cases you may feel that the 4 should be split up as 3 and 1; or 2 1 1. It is okay to answer in this fashion but do so sparingly.

When complete, add the column totals. As in the first set of answers high totals in the A column indicate **Vata;** the B column, **Pitta;** and C, **Kapha.**

The totals from this second half of the answer sheet will be smaller than the totals from the first, but are the totals from both answer sheets similar in proportion? Most participants will find this to be the case. If your totals do not match up relatively closely in terms of proportion then you have likely changed your mind since your first set of answers. (Are you Vata constitution?) Review your answers.

Keep in mind that whatever your Bodytype, it is okay: you are unique.

Keep in mind also that the score from the questionnaire may be skewed from an imbalance and need to be revised by common sense. Review the questionnaire after you have completed Session 7.

Review your taste preferences and aroma preferences. If your taste preferences are primarily for pacifying Vata, then your questionnaire should indicate Vata Constitution, or Vata imbalance.

Use your intuition as your first source of information and the questionnaire results as supplemental information. For example if you notice that some questions or statements for which you awarded high or low marks is a relatively new phenomenon in your life (for example dry skin) consider it an imbalance and delete the scoring from the total. See **Session 7**.

A Word of Caution and Encouragement

Even if you feel that you don't completely understand your constitution, or even if you are abysmally confused, you have made a start. Whatever your level of understanding there will be plenty of opportunity to refine this knowledge of constitution as the course progresses.

Some students understand their constitution immediately: others not so quickly. It took me quite a long time. Years later I am still learning how my physiology works.

If you wish to take a bit more time on this exercise consider the questionnaires once again, but don't turn it into work.

Paul Colver

Answer Sheet

Rate on a scale of 9 to 0, 9 being a definite yes, and 0 being a definite no. Do not use 4 or 5 as answers please.			
	A	B	C
1			
2			
3			
4			
5			
6			
7			
8			
9			
10			
11			
12			
13			
14			
15			
16			
17			
18			
19			
20			
21			
22			
23			
24			
25			
26			
27			
Total			

Award 4 to one space only. Or Use combinations of 3,2 or 1 sparingly.			
	A	B	C
1			
2			
3			
4			
5			
6			
7			
8			
9			
10			
11			
12			
13			
14			
15			
16			
17			
18			
19			
20			
21			
22			
23			
24			
25			
26			
27			
Total			

Reading and Websites

AUTHORS, TITLES AND WEBSITES FOR FURTHER STUDY

Anand, Margo: *The Art of Sexual Ecstasy.* www.margo-anand.com

Banchek, Linda: *The Ayurveda Cookbook: Cooking for Life.* The best cookbook I am aware of. Excellent quotes and understanding of Ayurvedic body types. The book could use more recipes. Vinegar is included in some of the recipes for Pitta, otherwise all seems well.

Bloomfield, Dr. Harold: *Making Peace with God,* from the series of books *Making Peace with Parents,...Your Self* etc. the last section of *Making Peace With God* presents a very clear account of what to look for, and to avoid, when choosing a meditation practice. Dr. Bloomfield's thinking and that of the author of *Enlightenment* (See Below) are strikingly consistent.

Chopra, Dr. Deepak: *Perfect Health; Perfect Digestion.* Dr. Chopra has done a great service in bringing a clear understanding of Ayurveda to the West. I highly recommend his early books which focus on Ayurveda.

Colver, Paul: *Before the Dawn.* www.paulcolver.info Though primarily written to touch the heart, the novel contains delightful passages that delve into the neurophysiology of consciousness.

Doige, Norman: MD, 2007 The Brain That Changes It-self—Stories of Personal Triumph from the Frontiers of Brain Science. Penguin Books; ISBN US 978-0-14-311310-2

Dossey, Dr. Larry: www.dosseydossey.com—*The Power of Prayer.* Though some of the early results from his research on the power of prayer have not been able to be easily replicated, his more current work regarding the effects of prayer on cultured cells is impossible to disregard.

Douillard, Dr. John: Invincible Athletics; Mind, Body, Sport www.lifespan.com Dr. Douillard's 20 year old program for athletics and fitness should by now be understood in every school, household and sports program in the world. While the nonsense of 'no pain—no gain' has spread like the Swine Flu, Dr. Douillard's brilliant approach to fitness has languished. It is a tragedy that his clear and insightful understanding of exercise and human physiology has largely been ignored.

Enlightenment, The Yoga Sutras of Patanjali, Translation and Commentary by MSI. ISBN #0 931783-17-8. An accurate and compelling commentary on the Vedic understanding of the neurophysiology of consciousness this work is also interesting in its congruence with Bloomfield's thinking. (See reference above)

Flanigan, Beverly, Forgiving Yourself: A Four Step Approach. Without self forgiveness we are suffering. Of all the things one can do for oneself forgiveness should be the first. An excellent book!

Gray, Dr. John: the Mars and Venus *series.* Gray's conceptions of men and women and their relationship potential are based in Vedic thought.

Hagelin, Dr. John: Renowned for being at the forefront of Quantum Physics, Dr. Hagelin's mammoth contributions and understandings of the Unified Field and its many applications is easily accessible on numerous websites. Google Hagelin for references to numerous sites and videos www.invincibledefense.org among them.

Hof, Lorne and Lucia: www.calllretreat.org. Modern day sages who are doing great things to bring enlightenment to many and increase the collective consciousness of our planet.

Ladd, Dr. Vasant: The Science of Self Healing. One of the earliest proponents of Ayurveda in the West Dr. Lad's writings and work has touched the lives of many.

Lonsdorf, Dr. Nancy: A Woman's Best Medicine and more recent *The Ageless Woman* www.vedichealth ct.org. Dr. Lonsdorf, a graduate of John Hopkins, is the world's most brilliant proponent of Maharishi Ayurveda.

Maharishi Mahesh Yogi: The Science of Being and the Art of Living; and *Commentary on the Bhagavad Gita: Chapters 1 to 6.* Both of these works cut through the quagmire of ignorance that engulfs much of the current thinking regarding evolution and consciousness in both India and the West. *The Commentary* is a work of genius.

Mate, Dr. Gabor www.drgabormate.com. Dr. Mate has currently written 2 books that are particularly interesting in their understanding of human physiology given that his education and career are from the traditional Western Medical model. Though he seems not to be familiar with Ayurveda he has yet reached many of Ayurveda's understandings regarding human physiology. Brilliant work.

Morrow, Pat: Beyond Everest: The Quest for 7 Summits www.patmorrow.com. Describes experiencing a flash of enlightenment on one of his climbs that energized him for months.

Nader, Dr. Tony: Human Physiology—Expression of Veda and Vedic Literature www.maharishitm.org. This is a monumental work that shows in detail the one to one correspondence of human physiology with the Unified Field, the Universe, Vedic Literature and the Ved. Every part of physiology is expressed in the Ved and every verse of the Ved has its counterpart in human physiology. Dr. Nader, a medical doctor and neurophysiologist, demonstrates how we are microcosms of the entire universe. In fact, we are created in the image of God.

Sharma, Dr. Hari: The Answer to Cancer, Freedom from Disease. Excellent books with both practical and theoretical info on how to avoid disease.

Sylvester, Richard: I Hope You Die Soon. www.richardsylvester.com. Uproariously happy with his enlightenment.

Tierra, Dr. Michael: The Way of Herbs www.planetherbs.com. Author and Herbalist with a comprehensive understand of herbology.

Tolle, Eckhart: The Power of Now www.eckharttolle.com. A modern day sage doing great things by awakening human consciousness.

Tam, Tom: Tom Tam Healing System www.tongrenshop.Com An interesting look at Chinese Medicine.

Vaidya Mishra: Raj Vaidya and Vedic Scholar extraordinaire. Vaidya Mishra during the past decade has brought the pristine wisdom of a 5000 year old family of Raj Vaidyas to North America through his teaching and consultations. www.vaidyamishra.com

Vasistha's Yoga, translated by Swami Venkatesananda, State University of New York Press. A voluminous and vibrant work replete with stories, and Vasistha's exhortations to Prince Rama as he leads him to enlightenment.

Wallace, Robert Keith, PhD. Dr. Wallace's research on, and description of, Transcendental Consciousness in the early 1970's continues to be the most overlooked of revolutionary scientists since Galileo. Pity. *The Physiology of Consciousness; The Maharishi Technology of the Unified Field: The Neurophysiology of Enlightenment.* Fairfield, Iowa: MIU Neuroscience Press, 1986.

Web sources of herb, heath information, research and articles.

www.bazaarofindia.com
www.mapi.com
www.theraj.com

About The Author

A former oilfield worker, shrimp boat deck hand, teacher, construction company owner, farmhand, management consultant, and recently, after years of trying, writer of the novel **Before the Dawn**, the first book of **The Satya Yuga Chronicles** which flowed forth with an intensity that was at times terrifying.

Later **The Aging Reversal Course** bubbled up, inspired by a lifelong interest in, and study of, Vedic thought.

Currently living in the City of Parksville, Vancouver Island the author is writing **Gaga in Zanzibar**, the story of a 60 year old man who after completing his first novel goes to Africa for three months to get away from words, falls into deep infatuation with a shining lass from Ireland, and lives out a long repressed Easy Rider fantasy by renting a motorcycle and touring the island of Zanzibar. His infatuation with the Irish lass prods the narrator to puzzle out his relationship with himself and with the five wonderful women who at various time graced his life.

Happily the father of two children they are often commend for following their dreams and reveling in life.

For work and amusement the author dabbles in politics, affordable housing, Vedic architecture, and teaches the course **Aging Reversal: An Ayurvedic Approach** at Vancouver Island University keeping his time fully occupied as he await (completely terrified) enlightenment.

Best wishes,
Paul Colver
Parksville, British Columbia

Endnotes

1   If you are not able to breathe comfortably through your nose because of an obstruction in one or both of nostrils see your doctor.

2   If there is no obstruction to the nasal passages but you find breathing this way challenging then introduce your body to this style of breathing very gradually. Most people make the switch easily but some do not. You may conclude that your body finds it easy and/or more useful to breathe through the mouth. One explanation for this is that breathing through the nose warms the air and breathing through the mouth cools the air. If your body requires you to breathe through the mouth this may be a good example of physiology having a need (to be cooled) that supersedes another need (the brain's need for oxygen). This is a classic case of two different systems within the body sending two conflicting messages.

Note also that there is a specific breathing exercise for drawing the breath over the surface of the tongue in order to cool the air. This exercise is discussed in Appendix P.

3   Though breathing through the nose makes use of the lower lungs it is not the full story on proper breathing. In some cases one should make full use of both the

lower and upper lungs. See Session 10: Vedic Exercise.)

4   Later in the course we will use this method of breathing during Session 10: Vedic Exercise. The numerous benefits to the physiology by breathing through the nose will be presented in later sessions.

5   Where the data of numerous studies is amalgamated and analyzed.

6   Our thoughts have power and influence the rebuilding and health of the body. See Session 5: Creating Physiology and Session 18: Quantum Mechanics and Human Physiology.

7   I remember the day before I left for my first week of treatment how while squatting to fill the truck tires my knees joints were on fire with pain. I returned after a week of PK with no pain in my joints. I've always believed that those PK sessions saved my health from completely collapsing.

8   This is not to say that if we are experiencing rage we pretend that we feel joy. See the Aggravation Exercise in Session 14.

9   As a caution regarding this understanding of how physiology is created we don't want to return to the Dark Age belief that healthy people are 'good' and sick people are 'bad'. From an Ayurvedic perspective if someone is ill it means they had a proclivity for that sickness and in order to deal with the challenge they need to support and strengthen the necessary systems within their physiology.

10   This is a bit of putting the cart before the horse as we will see when we discuss the releases of trauma in Session 15.

11   There is a notion in Ayurveda that the tastes should be introduced to the palette in the order of sweet, sour, salty, pungent, bitter and astringent. Eating the sweet food first makes sense in that bread, meat, milk etc. are heavy and require stronger digestion which is more likely to be available at the beginning of the meal.

12   Regarding weight management, one can work through all the diets under the sun but if each of the 6 tastes isn't satisfied weight management is likely to remain an immense challenge.

13   The people sharing the meal with you may not like your spice mixture and given what you have learned about the uniqueness of constitutions you by now probably understand their reticence. To deal with this situation place a ¼ teaspoon of your spice mix (or to suit) in ½ tbs of ghee in a fry pan and heat it just until you smell the pleasant aroma of the spices. See recipe for ghee in Appendix C.

14   Regarding moisture—Kapha constitution may tend to be oily whereas Pitta more often tends to sweat profusely.

15   This conception is vast and all encompassing and will be further clarified in Session 6: Individuality, Session 7: Creating Physiology and further Session 18: Quantum Mechanics and Human Physiology.

16   The Vedic conception of Vata, Pitta, and Kapha is vast and far more complex and all encompassing, as well

as fascinating than these few point above, and will be further explored throughout the course and particularly in Session 18: Quantum Mechanics and Human Physiology.

17   Please note that balance is not an equal division of Vata, Pitta and Kapha. Balance is having the three doshas in proper proportions, and properly located within our body, as initially established.

18   Pitta!

19   Vaidya Mishra (see Reading and Websites) has a powdered DGL (diglicerated licorice) which tastes good in this tea. DGL has most of the sugar removed.

20   Fruit peelings, similar to brown rice and the like, are thought to be difficult to digest. Your body's intelligence is your best guide.

21   Cloves are pungent, but the taste, as they are digested, becomes sweet and the effect of them is to open the various channels without heating up the physiology. They are a great way for people with hot constitutions to satisfy their need for a pungent taste.

22   Combining 2 grains increases the chances of making complete protein available.

23   Ayurveda recommends that vegetables be cooked until you can easily stick a fork into them.

24   See Appendix C.

25   3½ percent is not the whole milk. Do you remember the milk from the 50's in the glass bottles? It was about 15 or 20 percent cream.

26   Note that an early time of day for the evening meal is recommended. At varying times of the year the evening meal may be taken in either the Vata or Kapha

time of day. Ie, vata time of day in summer, early kapha time of day in winter.

27   While I enjoy summer, by the end of it I am dunking my head in ice water and opening the freezer and joyfully breathing in cool air. Is this abnormal behavior? Possibly, but how much more so is it to have a raging Pitta imbalance?

28   So far our costs have been minimal—spices and oils and organic food, but a trip to a Pancha Karma center will change all that. See www.theraj.com.

29   Stryker and Wallace, Regarding a reduction in biological aging through an Ayurvedic treatment program. Paper at the International Congress of Psychosomatic Medicine, Chicago, September 1985.

30   The ghee prep is not suitable for all constitutions (particularly Kapha) and the amounts should be adjusted depending on the constitution (less for Vata and more for Pitta). If you are going to try this on your own be very cautious: use very small amounts to begin. And do not be involved in any vigorous activity.

31   Yogi's burning off remaining karma.

32   Do you know that the average life expectancy of a professional football player is 56 years? Are you going to listen to me or Knute Rockney? If you don't feel well, then rest.

33   In fact, there are areas they do not seem to stretch though I practice only two dozen of 84,000 postures.

34   Sleep with the crown of the head facing East as the gravity of the morning sun pulls various goodies to the brain.

35   In order to understand this unknown called Life some inquisitive folks have resorted to autopsying corpses in order to find what is missing. All the parts are intact: what is missing is Life.

36   Turkey and chicken, later in the digestive process, have a cooling effect.

37   Ayurveda frowns on foods that are difficult to digest. For example brown rice though more nutritious than white is harder to digest. Ayurveda considers good digestion to be an absolute necessity for vibrant health and in cases of weak digestion recommends less nutritious, but more easily digestible food.

38   There is nothing esoteric about Marmas. For example the thymus gland which has blood vessels, nerves, and is responsible for governing the lymphatic system is a Marma.

39   A caution in practicing Pranayama is that it should be gentle and not forced, and it requires your full, easy focus. Probably a maximum practice time of 5 minutes is most suitable and it is best practiced prior to meditation or prayer, with a rest period after. It is not suitable practiced before sleep or during activity. (See Appendix P)

40   Have you found any areas of your body that cry out for extra attention during Abhyanga? You may have found a Marma. Please recall or reread the cautions about which direction to massage the joints, as energy of the Marmas spin correctly in one direction only; the same as the solar system and the galaxies.

41   We will refer to research by Keith Wallace on this concept in our next session.

42 Patrick Morrow, in his book describing an experience he had climbing a mountain, is an excellent description of transcendence.

43 Vedic Medicine with its understanding of sound has additional insight into healing bones. See Session 18: Quantum Mechanics and Human Physiology.

44 'Ownership', as so often preached, does not mean that when one is seriously ill the reason is that we willed the illness. Ownership means we could have focused more on strengthening our physiology.

45 The Professional football player's description of full awareness of the entire playing field during a crucial game is a remarkable example of full, undivided attention while immersed in activity.

46 This is not to say that we should willy-nilly dredge up traumatic memories.

47 This is not to say that activity may not be performed in this silence but that is the subject of another book that someone other than I will write.

48 Interestingly enough this is a common approach in the West. Note the experiences reported by tri-athletes, runners, mountaineers and other uber athletes. At levels of extreme exhaustion the body is sometimes forced into deep rest.

49 A white sticky toxic substance produced during poor digestion.

50 Though perfect digestion would seem to be the ultimate basis for health and aging reversal there are other prerequisites. They too are part of human physiology but far beyond the scope of this course. I of course am currently interested in a focus on perfect

digestion and letting a wiser teacher than I will appear in your life to teach you these more advance aspects of human physiology. Make sure and phone me so I can tag along.

51 Often meditation techniques arise when a traveler is given what are purported to be the keys to the kingdom from a fish seller in some exotic corner of the world and then the traveler returns to the West, writes a book, and begins (often with great sincerity) the Meditation of the Holy Fish Seller.

52 I use the quotation marks to indicate that these words are not an accurate description of the idea they attempt to describe. The moral of the story is to find a meditation teacher you can trust on the basis of what western science has to report regarding the effects of the technique.

53 See Mapi and Mishra websites.

54 Available to each of us in order that we can contact, enliven and make manifest the qualities of the Unmanifest. See tm.org

55 Validity: that what is purportedly being measured is in fact what is being measured. Reliability: that the experiment may be replicated with the same results.

56 In my view Being must first be enlivened in human consciousness. I don't say that a person should not act when they have the urge to bring about change. I do say that a person not at peace within themselves is an odd person to try to create world peace. Nonetheless the unfolding Universe is a mysterious business and in that regard I encourage people to work at whatever best suits their sense of Dharma.